For my wife,
MARISOL,
who still insists I snore

Laugh, and the world laughs with you;
snore, and you sleep alone.

— ANTHONY BURGESS, *novelist*

SNORE NO MORE!

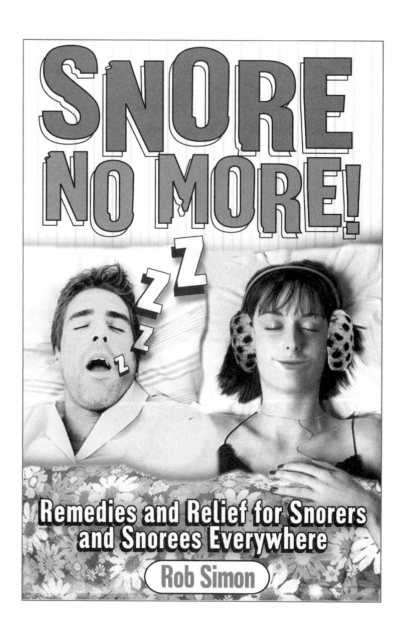

SNORE NO MORE!

Remedies and Relief for Snorers and Snorees Everywhere

Rob Simon

**Andrews McMeel
Publishing**

Kansas City

05 06 07 08 09 RR4 10 9 8 7 6 5 4 3 2 1

Simon, Rob
 Snore, no more! : remedies and relief for snorers and
 snorees everywhere / Rob Simon.
    p. cm.
 ISBN 0-7407-5036-4
   1. Snoring—Popular works. I. Title.
 RA786.3.S56 2005
 616.2'09—dc22

                                     2004066008

Book design by Pete Lippincott

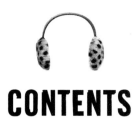

CONTENTS

CONTENTS

Appendixes

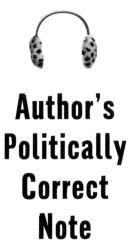

Author's Politically Correct Note

IN THIS BOOK, I HAD MANY CHOICES when using the third-person pronoun to describe a snorer. I decided not to alternate between "he" and "she," as this is a book, not a Ping-Pong game. I decided not to use "he/she" as it looks silly. Besides, there is no such thing as a he/she, except in certain parts of the world. I will not use "their" as this is a cop-out and causes all kinds of other grammatical problems. Nor will I use "it" even though snorers sound nonhuman. I will use "he." Since men are twice as likely as women to snore, not only is this politically correct, it's also scientifically accurate.

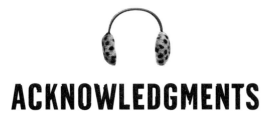

ACKNOWLEDGMENTS

I WANT TO THANK ALL THE DOCTORS, researchers, books, patients, snorers, snorees, and Web sites that have taught me more than I ever wanted to know about how my nose does and doesn't work. This book is filled with their information.

I tip my hat to the Scandinavian countries, which seem to have done most of the research on why people snore and how they can stop. Also, thanks to the Japanese, the British, and the Australians, who are fascinated by snoring. I marvel at American ingenuity for creating and selling snoring cures like snake oil (this, by the way, actually might cure snoring if you gargled with it). I owe a huge debt of gratitude to the Internet, which empowered me to do most of my research from the privacy of my study. Thanks, World Wide Web.

I want to thank my parents for their prosnoring genetics, and especially my father, who is a one-man search engine for health information. To my brother, thanks for your support. I want to thank my children, Ben and Claire, for their patience in suffering through my late-night noises as a writer

ACKNOWLEDGMENTS

and a snorer. To Julie Burton, thank you for your early belief and ongoing advice.

And to my wife, Marisol, who is my muse for writing and life, as always, thank you.

INTRODUCTION

"FINALLY, A CURE FOR SNORING!"

How many times have you heard that?

If you are a snorer, you have seen this claim on the stop-snoring Web sites, books, e-mail offers, pillows, devices, straps, sprays, and herbal cures that you have tried—but nothing seems to work.

"Finally, a cure for snoring that *works*!" If the cure truly worked, they wouldn't have to advertise it, right? Well, in addition to yourself, the 90 million other snorers would be flocking to the cure like moths to a light—a very bright light. A very bright light with lots of good moth food and good things for moths to drink.

"Finally, a cure for snoring that works—*guaranteed*!" If there really was ONE guaranteed cure, we snorers wouldn't even need this book.

On the other side of the bed, if you sleep—or attempt to sleep—with a snorer, these final cures for snoring have something else in common besides their futility: Except for earplugs and second bedrooms, virtually nothing is for *you*—the person who is *really* suffering, the one trying to live with the snorer—the "snoree."

This is perhaps the first book for snorers *and* snorees everywhere, providing remedies for this noisy epidemic, and comic relief when those remedies fall short.

This is not your typical self-help book. Sure, it will help the snorer search for a cure—assuming he thinks he has a problem in the first place. More often than not it's the snorees who are motivated to solve the problem—even though it's not theirs to begin with. They're the ones who need relief and a good night's sleep, and if not that, at least empathy and perhaps a good laugh. That's why for the snoree, it's not a self-help book, it's a "*you*-need-help" book. Buy it for, and give it to, someone you "love."

This book will help you understand why people snore; find a cure; and at least live with and laugh at the problem. It may even save your relationship—as writing this saved mine. Perhaps one of the many cures included here *will* work, or perhaps you'll find something that's a livable compromise. Either way, I hope the grin and tonic of laughter will lighten the burden of lost sleep along the way.

If neither the chuckles nor the cures work, you can always throw this book at your snoring partner's head, which usually *does* stop them from snoring (but not too hard or they'll stop breathing, too). That's why it's better to buy my hefty book now and not wait until it gets trimmed down for *Reader's Digest.* You shouldn't wait for the book to be made into a reality TV show or movie either. Can you even imagine a movie on snoring? *Finally, Snore No More,* starring Dustin Hoffman as the snorer and Glenn Close as the homicidal snoree.

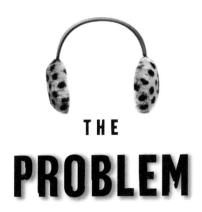

THE
PROBLEM

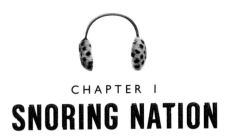

CHAPTER I
SNORING NATION

MORE THAN 90 MILLION AMERICANS SNORE every night. And for many snorers blissfully grinding their gears while they sleep, there is someone next to them—a snoree—who suffers through a sleepless night.

Wake up, America, you are a snoring nation, and this book is for you.

Maybe it's you who snores. Maybe it's your husband or wife. Or maybe it's your partner or your roommate who snores. It could be your kids. Or maybe it's your dog. Yes, even pets snore, although it's difficult to tell when tropical fish snore, since it all sounds like gurgling.

If you snore or if you try to sleep next to a snorer, then this book is for you.

It's not just an American thing—nearly 40 percent of the adult world snores. That's almost 2 billion snorers and at least

2 billion snorees, depending upon how many people sleep in the same room, house, or hut.

They are snoring (*ibiki*) in Tokyo. They are snoring (*ronflement*) in Paris. They are snoring (*schnarchen*) in Berlin. They are snoring (*xpan*) in Moscow. They are snoring (*roncando*) in Caracas. They are especially snoring in the Netherlands (*snurken, snorken, knorren, ronken, stertor, reutelen, rochelen, geronk, gesnurk*).

I may have trouble with phrase books, and the languages may be different, but the sound of snoring needs no translation. Snorers and snorees of the world, unite!

(**TABLE 1**)

SNORING TRANSLATED AROUND THE WORLD
(WEBSTER'S ONLINE DICTIONARY)

Language	Word for Snore or Snoring	Translation
English (American)	snore, stertor, rhonchus, snark, saw logs, drive pigs to market	Grrrgchroar
English (British)	I say, snoring	Grrrgchroar
English (Canadian)	snoring, eh?	Grrrgchroar
Danish	*snorken*	Grrrgchroar

SNORING NATION

Language	Word for Snore or Snoring	Translation
Dutch	snurken, snorken, knorren, ronken, stertor, reutelen, rochelen, geronk, gesnurk	Grrrgchroar
French	ronflement, ronflez, vrombir	Grrrgchroar
German	schnarchen	Grrrgchroar
Hebrew	י נ רח ת נ	Grrrgchroar
Hungarian	horkoló, horkolás, hortyogó, hortyogás	Grrrgchroar
Italian	russamento	Grrrgchroar
Japanese	ibiki, kansui (accomplishment, brackish water, flooding, sprinkling, submerge)	Grrrgchroar
Portuguese	ronco (bellow, growl, grunt) ressono	Grrrgchroar
Pig Latin	oringsnay	RoarGrrrgchsnay
Real Latin	stertere	Grrrgchroar
Romanian	sforãitor, sforãialã, horcãit, horãit	Grrrgchroar
Russian	храп	Grrrgchroar
Spanish	roncando	Grrrgchroar
Swedish	snarka, snarkning	Grrrgchroar

continued

TABLE I *Continued*

Language	Word for Snore or Snoring	Translation
Ukranian	хропіння (khropinnia)	Grrrgchroar
Welsh	*chwyrniad* (snarl)	Grrrgchroar

If you live in any of the countries in Table 1, or even if your country is not in Table 1, and you snore or live with a snorer, this book is for you. If you would like your country to be listed in Table 1, please write to the author (rob@snorebook.com).

As a word, "snoring" first appeared in English literature in the early 1300s. It comes from the Middle English *snoren,* "to snort," and from the Old English *fnora,* "to sneeze." In Turkey, snoring comes from a word that means carpet sweeper or hell. Hmmmm, I think the Turks have it right.

As a concept, snoring was around in the Garden of Eden—why do you think Eve kicked Adam out? The whole snake-apple thing was overstated. Adam was the original snorer (the original "original sin") because men are twice as likely to snore as women. Overweight men are even more likely—especially overweight men over forty who sleep on their backs, drink beer, smoke, snack before going to bed, and only exercise by flipping the remote. Did I leave any men out?

Eve, and women of the world—this book is for you.

And since men sleep with men on ships, this book is for some men, too. Sailors, here is the word "snoring" in semaphore.

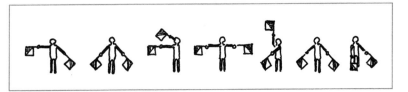

"Snoring" in Semaphore

Snoring is everywhere. On the Internet, the word "snoring" is searched an average of 1,220 times per day, while "stop snoring" is only searched 323 times per day. If you do the math, does that mean 897 people are searching to *start* snoring? No, they are searching for specific cures. "Snoring surgery" is searched thirty-five times per day. "Snoring pillows" are searched eleven times per day. "Snoring spray" is searched thirteen times. "Snoring dogs" is searched six times per day.

It is entirely possible that male dogs over the age of six (forty-two in human years) that eat too much and don't exercise are more likely to snore. If female dogs had thumbs, they'd search the Internet for cures, too.

Pet owners, and pets with thumbs, you are part of our snoring nation, and this book is for you.

On a serious note, snoring can be the symptom of a potentially life-threatening condition—sleep apnea, or stoppage of breathing. While this book will address some noncritical sleepless conditions, if you have sleep apnea, seek proper medical attention.

This book is for the perpetrators and the victims of what is now fashionably called "antisocial snoring." My definition: *Antisocial snoring, while not life-threatening, does threaten the quality of life of both the snorer and the snoree, especially when the snoree threatens the snorer's life.*

If you haven't guessed by now, I am an antisocial snorer and my wife is the recipient of my antisocial activity.

To find a cure for my snoring, I read almost every book, visited almost every Web site, and consulted every doctor and sleep specialist I could find. I followed everyone's advice. I lost weight, stopped drinking, stopped smoking (before I even started), changed sleeping positions, changed pillows, un-deviated my deviated septum, dilated my sinuses with acid, reshaped my palate with lasers, irrigated my nasal passages, used herbal sprays, tried bizarre mouth and chin devices only sold through the Internet, and removed my uvula before I even knew what or where it was.

Today, I snore no more. Well, sort of. I still snore a little, but it's manageable. All the remedies I experimented with do work—not the same for everyone, but they do work.

Trying these cures and my wife's patience is what led me to write this book. However, the more cures I tried, the more I continued to snore, and the more frustrated we became, until suddenly a new sound started emerging from the bedroom—laughter. Snoring became funny for both of us. Moreover, we discovered that by laughing about my snoring we were able to acknowledge its impact on our life as a couple. I was able to "own the problem," search for a cure, and write a book in which I actually use "own the problem" in a sentence.

I'm a self-help guru now.

Aside from an occasional whack in the head or sleeping in the next room, laughter truly became the best medicine. Humor—and some surgeries on my nose—saved our relationship. Because, let's face it, snoring only becomes a problem when it's in a relationship. Does anyone who sleeps alone try to stop snoring? Do they even *know* they snore? No way. What's that old adage? "If a man snores in the forest, and there's no one to hear it, was there a sound?"

Who cares, snoring's not philosophy, it's noise. If you don't believe me, just ask Mrs. Sartre.

CHAPTER 2

WHY DO PEOPLE SNORE?

WHY DO PEOPLE SNORE? Simply stated, they can't help themselves.

Blame It on the Soft Palate

Snoring is caused when the soft tissues in the back of the mouth and nose relax during sleep, and then, with every incoming breath, flap like a sail in the wind, or vibrate like a cicada rubbing its legs together, or both. In musical terms, these soft tissues act like the reed of a clarinet or oboe, only instead of creating harmony they create cacophony.

The part of the mouth causing this ruckus is known as the soft palate. It's the archway at the back of the throat where the uvula literally hangs out—the little boxing bag of flesh that dangles from the roof of your mouth and always rattles in cartoons when someone yells.

So why *do* some people snore and others don't?

Half of the adults in the world have enough space to breathe through their noses and throats while sleeping without making noise, but the other half do not. When certain conditions (which I'll explain later) reduce this space by only a little, a person is forced to breathe through his mouth, and snoring happens. Oh, and by the way, nose-breathers can be snorers, too.

Here's the medical view of what happens by breathing through the mouth: (a) The tongue collapses backward, pushing the uvula against the back of the throat; (b) the relaxed tissues along the soft palate vibrate; and now (c) everything in the back of the mouth shakes, rattles, and rolls, like driving over the wake-me-up slots on the shoulder of a highway.

It's not a pretty picture no matter how you slice it. (See Figure 2.)

There are two reasons people don't snore while walking, shopping, working, hunting, or sneaking overdue videos into the drop-off box hoping the clerks won't know the difference. First, when people are awake they normally breathe through their noses and not their mouths. Second, the soft tissues need to *relax* before they can flap and vibrate to make noise, and that only happens when people sleep or go to their kids' school concerts.

FIGURE 2

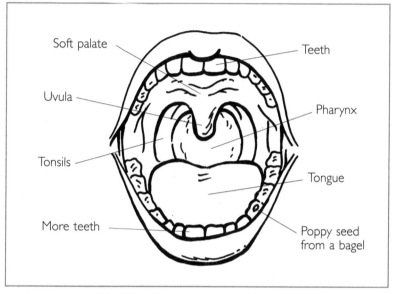

Soft palate

Teeth

Uvula

Pharynx

Tonsils

Tongue

More teeth

Poppy seed
from a bagel

A Not-So-Pretty Picture of Snoring

The Margin for Error in a Nose

To understand how easy it is to snore, one must first understand the margin for error in a nose. A nose contains two
narrow passages, or nostrils, through which we breathe. At
the back of each nostril is an even narrower space called the
nasal valve. This valve governs airflow into our lungs and is
only one-tenth of an inch wide—thinner than a dime—so it

has a lot of work to do when you compare its size to the amount of air it manages.

Each valve is surrounded by even tinier blood vessels. When these blood vessels swell, they put pressure on the valves. This restricts breathing and forces one to breathe through the mouth, and that's when the trouble starts.

Clearly then, *anything* that causes these blood vessels to swell, or entices the soft tissues to constrict or relax, will create or exacerbate a snoring condition. In fact, the very act of lying down causes water to accumulate around these infamous blood vessels and makes them engorge. You see, we don't even have a chance. Snoring is one of the few problems left we can legitimately blame on something else. (Aha! That means we don't "own the problem" after all; we merely rent it.)

The Conditions for Snoring

For people who don't have enough space in their noses and are prone to snoring, here are the common conditions that will make them snore:

- Sleeping on your back, which can force your tongue to the back of your mouth where either it vibrates or it pushes the uvula into vibrating, or both

- Using a pillow that is too large and moves your head forward, constricting your throat

- Drinking alcohol, which makes everything relax

- Taking sleeping pills, cold medicine, or any medication with sedatives or some antihistamines that irritate the throat

- Smoking, which narrows the passageways, and irritates the throat and nasal valves

- Getting pregnant (not recommended for men), which increases the blood flow and narrows the nasal passages

- Eating a large meal before bedtime

- Being overweight

- Sleeping with a tie or noose around your neck

In fact, there is nothing more problematic for snoring than extra poundage. When a person is overweight, his tongue, neck, face, and soft palate get flabby, too. The heft of your uvula, tongue, and throat is such an important factor in restricting the intake of air, going on a diet is the first thing doctors recommend to stop snoring.

But wait, there's more. Even a person with restricted nasal passages who is *not* breathing through his mouth can still snore. Why? Because he is breathing harder through his nose, and this extra force can still cause the soft tissues in the back of the mouth to vibrate.

There's even more to the nightmare. When we're awake, it's normal to breathe through both nostrils and nasal valves. When we sleep, however, these tiny passages take turns. This reduces the margin for error by half and makes mouth breathing during sleep that much more necessary and likely.

It Can Be Hereditary

Who's your daddy, and does he snore? There are hereditary conditions and physical changes to your "airflow infrastructure" that might make things even worse. People with a collar size of more than seventeen and a half inches—fat-necked football players and refrigerator repairmen, for instance—are more likely to snore because an oversized neck squeezes down on the throat. A person also can be born with an unusually shaped jaw or mouth that restricts the airflow. A broken nose, deviated septum, nasal polyps, and overly large tonsils and adenoids can narrow or restrict the airflow infrastructure. Allergies and other respiratory ailments might also create a condition for snoring.

Men Snore More, Old Men Snore Even More

Studies have shown that both gender and age affect snoring. Snoring is twice as common in men as in women, and it doesn't take a sleep specialist to figure out why. Men are more likely to have bulky tissues (fat necks, tongues, throats, etc.) and load themselves up with snore-inducing habits such as drinking, smoking, overeating, and sleeping on their backs a lot—like whales in odd places. However, after women reach menopause, they catch up to the guys a bit and begin snoring because they now have less estrogen. (Higher quantities of estrogen stimulate breathing and thus reduce snoring.)

As people age, they also are more likely to snore. Nearly 80 percent of people over the age of sixty snore. As we age, we gain weight and lose muscle tone, two prime conditions for snoring.

When you add up all the conditions that lead to snoring, it's a miracle the whole world doesn't snore.

Dangerous Snoring: Obstructive Sleep Apnea (OSA)

On a serious note, snoring can be a symptom of something more dangerous than an angry bedfellow. When the soft tissues relax or constrict so severely that they collapse, this can actually obstruct the oral passageway and cause a person to stop breathing. When this happens for ten seconds or more, it is known as obstructive sleep apnea. When a person's airflow is reduced by more than half, it's known as a hypopnea.

People with obstructive sleep apneas might stop breathing dozens of times an hour or hundreds of times a night (usually preceded by a snorting sound or snore). One woman measured at a sleep clinic was waking up 215 times an hour! This becomes dangerous when these apneas and hypopneas accumulate and create a drop of oxygen in the blood supply, sometimes to alarmingly low levels.

Over time, or as the apneas increase in frequency and strength, oxygen deprivation accumulates and can cause cells to malfunction or become permanently damaged. Serious health problems may follow, such as elevated blood pressure, increased chance of stroke or heart attack, increased blood pressure in the vessels of the lungs, irregular heartbeats, fatigue, depression, loss of sex drive, impotence, and uncontrollable sleep attacks known as narcolepsy.

At the very least, these apneas lead to irritability and sleep deprivation that decrease mental sharpness and alertness. This can pose serious dangers while driving, operating heavy equipment, or balancing your checkbook.

If you think the person next to you might have sleep apnea, he should see a doctor or sleep specialist, since it may be a symptom of something more serious than "antisocial" snoring. (Please see "Is It Apnea?" on page 20.) The doctor most likely will require your snoring partner to take an overnight polysomnogram sleep study. This procedure scientifically measures the frequency and severity of the apneas and hypopneas.

Upper Airway Resistance Syndrome (UARS)

If you have many of the symptoms of obstructive sleep apnea, i.e., drowsiness during the day without the dangerous loss of oxygen during the night, you may suffer from upper airway resistance syndrome. It is halfway between antisocial snoring and obstructive sleep apnea. You most likely will show up "negative" for apneas on any overnight polysomnogram sleep studies, but your snoree partner is absolutely "positive" you snore like a horse.

After taking a polysomnogram, I was diagnosed with UARS or "mini-apneas" as the doctor called them. I liked the sound of UARS over mini-apneas. Mini-apneas sounded cute, like getting the goosebumps, but UARS sounded serious, like a real condition. I wasn't just snoring, I had UARS! I felt vindicated.

I began to use UARS as an excuse to get out of doing things. "Sorry. I can't take care of your cat while you're on vacation, I have UARS." "No thank you, I'll pass on the mushroom-eggplant soup—you know I have UARS." "No, I can't attend your fund-raising event. I have UARS. In fact, I'm going to a UARS fund-raising event that same evening." I thought I would become the poster child for UARS.

However, I got mini-sympathy (for my mini-apneas) for only about a week. Sooner or later I would have to treat my UARS and stop my snoring madness.

IS IT APNEA?

If the person next to you demonstrates any or all of the following symptoms, he may have sleep apnea and should see a doctor or sleep specialist.

- Does his own snoring wake him up?

- Does he feel like he can't catch his breath or breathe comfortably while sleeping?

- Does he wake in the morning with a headache?

- Does he wake feeling tired even after he's had a complete night's sleep?

- Is he irritable during the day?

- Is he likely to nap during the day?

- Does he ever close his eyes or doze unexpectedly, for example while driving, during a meeting, or in conversation?

CHAPTER 3

THE SOUND OF SNORING

FROM THE SNORER'S SIDE OF THE BED, the sound of snoring sounds like denial:

"What sound? I didn't hear anything."

From the snoree's side of the bed, the sound that cuts through the night and ruins the best of sleeps is almost impossible to describe. Snorees resort to using similes such as:

"You sound like a foghorn."

"You sound like a chainsaw."

"You sound like a garbage disposal."

"You sound like a spoon stuck in a garbage disposal."

"You sound like a chainsaw trying to remove a spoon stuck in a garbage disposal, while a plumber in the background roots with a foghorn."

Sound familiar? If none of these similes work, then you should try metaphors.

"Your snoring is my worst nightmare."

"Your snoring is a train wreck."

"Your snoring is a power tool on steroids."

If similes and metaphors still don't work, then you should try insults and threats.

"You are a snoring monkey [insert rhinoceros, elephant, dog, or other animal of your choice]."

"If you don't stop snoring, I will hunt you down and kill you like the snoring monkey [or rhinoceros, elephant, dog, or other animal you have chosen] that you are."

Snorees search for better ways to describe snoring because snoring is not only a sound, it's a rude awakening. Snorees naively believe that the more accurately they describe the sound, the more it will wake their snoring partners from their complacency. It's a desperate plea for help: Only the perfect description will make snorers understand how loud, how rude, how preternaturally dangerous, their snoring is, and that understanding could lead to a cure.

Here's how Mark Twain described Big Jim's snore in *Tom Sawyer Abroad*.

> Jim begun to snore—soft and blubbery at first, then a long rasp, then a stronger one, then a half a dozen horrible ones like the last water sucking down the plug-hole of a bath-tub, then the same with more power to it, and some big coughs and snorts flung in, the way a cow does that is choking to death; and

when the person has got to that point he is at his level best, and can wake up a man that is in the next block with a dipperful of loddanum in him, but can't wake himself up although all that awful noise of his'n ain't but three inches from his own ears.

To the discerning snoree, there are three components to a snore: loudness, tenor, and frequency.

Loudness

The loudness of a snore is determined by a mixture of many factors: the size of the snorer's nasal passages, the depth of his breathing, and the amount of soft tissue in the back of the throat causing all the noise. Even petite, sweet-looking people can emit ungodly snores disproportionate to their size if their internal acoustics are right.

(**FACT**)

Gunfighter John Wesley Hardin was so infuriated by a man snoring loudly in the hotel room next to him that he fired several bullets through the bedroom wall—first waking the snorer, then killing him.

Regardless of how you describe the sound, all snorees would agree that snoring is loud. In fact, snoring is perhaps one of the most quantifiably annoying sounds on earth. (See Table 2.)

(**TABLE 2**)

MOST ANNOYING SOUNDS ON EARTH

Sound	Decibel Level
Silence—the threshold of hearing	0 dBs
The level at which sleep is disturbed	30 dBs
Quiet conversation with your mother	40 dBs
Quiet conversation with your father	45 dBs
Office noise	50 dBs
Garbage disposal	60 dBs
Snoring	60–80 dBs
Heavy truck traffic	80 dBs
Jackhammer on concrete	82 dBs
Loud Snoring	90 dBs
New York City subway	100 dBs
Chainsaw	100 dBs

Sound	Decibel Level
747 jet taking off	110 dBs
World's Loudest Snore—Alan Myatt	112.8 dBs
Ouch—the threshold of pain	135 dBs
Uh-oh. Death occurs	155 dBs

(FACT)

In California, a woman was fined $135 for disturbing the peace because of her snoring.

Tenor

In addition to the loudness of snoring, there is the tenor, or the texture, of each snore. A good snorer is able to compose a symphony of snores every night. A discerning snoree is able to classify each of these snores as a gourmand appreciates wines.

The Wheeze. The wheeze is an even, light-bodied snore with a soft beginning and finish. This snore, with its gentle yet constant texture, is like the incessant and irritating hum of fluorescent bulbs. It lasts all night, constant and flat, and therein lies its terror. While not exceptionally loud, it makes up for it in annoyance and consistency.

The Snort. The snort is a powerful snore: short, loud, and frightening. It's a sudden gasp for breath, as if the snorer is drowning or has been shot in the throat. It usually arrives with the first sign of sleep and, in fact, can signal sleep as a pig snorts before dinner. While sometimes it is a singular act, be warned: It typically returns several times throughout the evening when the snorer naturally awakens and falls back to sleep. Or it can be paired with any of the other snoring sounds.

The Darth Vader. If this were a wine, it would be described as having a spicy and medium-bodied bouquet. It starts and ends with a sinister flourish. Akin to the wheeze, this snore is consistent with every breath, but with more force—from the dark side. Its signature: a robust, bass-toned sound, as if the snorer is James Earl Jones laboring with every breath, sucking air through an ill-fitting mask and a corroded windpipe.

The Gargle. The most common of snores, the gargle sounds as if the snorer is sleeping and breathing with a cup of mouthwash perpetually stuck in the back of his throat. With every incoming breath, this full-bodied snore has a strong finish with overtones of power tools. It is often spelled as "grrrggccchh."

The Whistle. The rarest of snores, as popularized by the Three Stooges, it is the only one made upon exhaling, not inhaling. Piquant and peppery, its playfulness disguises its true annoying character.

Frequency

Some people snore all night, every night. Some snore only when they first fall asleep. Others snore only when conditions are ripe, creating a nightly air of uncertainty: Will he or won't he tonight? In fact, this expectation of sound can be almost as exasperating as the sound itself.

While the frequency of snoring will vary from snorer to snorer and night to night, most snorees will agree it only takes one time per evening to disrupt a good night's sleep.

Consequences

While the antisocial snorer rarely loses any sleep over it, the snoree loses a lot. One research study in Sweden concluded that over time, a snoree sleeping next to a loud snorer actually experiences hearing loss. The Mayo Clinic recently demonstrated that the average snoree loses more than one hour of sleep every night. Even one hour of lost sleep can lead to an assortment of daytime consequences for the snoree ranging from annoying to extreme:

- Anger and resentment toward the snorer
- Chronic fatigue

- Headaches

- Irritability

- Forgetfulness

- Loss of sex drive

- Loss of motor skills, like driving

- Loss of having sex while driving or motoring

(FACT)

Sleep deprivation causes more than $12 billion worth of automobile accidents every year. The U.S. Commission on Sleep Disorders found that drowsiness was a factor in 50 percent of all traffic accidents and 36 percent of all fatal accidents.

(FACT)

Sleep deprivation was a significant factor in the *Exxon Valdez* oil tanker spill, the *Challenger* space shuttle crash, and the nuclear disaster at Chernobyl.

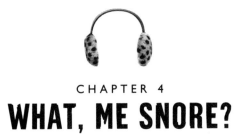

CHAPTER 4

WHAT, ME SNORE?

WHY DO PEOPLE DENY THEY SNORE?

Let's state the obvious. Snoring of the antisocial variety is only a problem when it's in a relationship. No relationship, no snoring. No single person ever woke up in the morning and said, "What was that awful noise last night? I must have been snoring. Gotta do something about that today *before* I get into a relationship that I care about."

In fact, most single people don't even know they snore unless they "snore around," in which case they are told they snore, but they just don't care.

Mark Twain said it best in *Tom Sawyer Abroad:* "There ain't no way to find out why a snorer can't hear himself snore." Many other famous people snore (see Table 3).

Hearing your own snore is like trying to watch yourself sneeze in the mirror. (Just as you are about to sneeze, your eyes automatically close, making it impossible to see

(**TABLE 3**)

FAMOUS PEOPLE WE KNOW SNORE

Famous Person
Elizabeth Taylor
The Three Stooges
Sir John Falstaff (in *Henry IV* by William Shakespeare)
Fat Joe in *The Pickwick Papers* by Charles Dickens
Winston Churchill
Franklin Delano Roosevelt
Benito Mussolini
Regis Philbin
The Sundance Kid
Frank Gifford
Morley Safer
Howard Stern
George Washington
Abraham Lincoln
Beau Brummell
Every overweight president: Taft, Harding, McKinley

FAMOUS PEOPLE WE SUSPECT SNORE BUT DIDN'T ASK

Famous Person
Orson Welles
Roseanne Barr

Famous Person
Bill Clinton
Pliny the Elder
Dustin Hoffman
Pliny the Younger
Raymond Burr
Nikita Khruschev
Anyone named Pliny
Goofy
Barbra Streisand

anything.) And just as you are about to snore, you fall into a deep sleep, making it impossible to *hear* anything. When you awaken, the snoring is already aural history. It's a blissful state of ignorance.

That is, until someone you care about (or not) sleeps next to you and hears the rumble. One day you're a happy sleeper, the next you're a guilty snorer. The rude awakening to the snoree, however, is swift compared to the often drawn-out consciousness raising that must occur for the snorer to admit his culpability.

Typically, a snoree will "live" with the snoring and not say anything for a period of time that can be days, weeks, or months depending upon the snoree's patience and tolerance for lost sleep. When the snoree reaches a breaking point, however, pent-up frustration can lead to a classic rookie mistake. In the morning a sleep-deprived snoree may say accusingly, "You were snoring last night and it woke me up!" This immediately puts the snorer on the defensive. Cornered, his only retort is, "What, *me* snore? *You* must have been dreaming."

This confrontation leaves both parties wounded. The snoree feels violated, dismissed, and sleep-deprived, while the snorer feels rested of course, and as if he has shacked up with a lunatic.

Before attempting to resolve the situation and search for a cure, the snoring partner must be encouraged to accept responsibility and "ownership of the problem." Only then will the snorer attempt to look for a cure. Why should a snorer fix something that he thinks isn't even broken?

The Nine Stages of Snoring Denial (NSSD)

The snoree would do better to learn the NSSD scale to determine where her snoring partner falls in the continuum from denial to ownership of the problem. (See Table 4.) Since most snorers are men, these stages bring out some of man's most "endearing" traits such as self-aggrandizement and capacity for fabrication. (For a complete list of man's most endearing traits, please read the *Iliad* by Homer or spend fifteen minutes with Donald Trump.)

TABLE 4

NINE STAGES OF SNORING DENIAL

Stage	Typical Snorer Responses
1 Indignation	I don't snore. Period. Never have, never will.
2 Incredulity	What, me snore? You must have been dreaming. You probably heard something else, like the neighbor opening the garage door.
3 Projection	*You* must be a light sleeper. No one else has ever mentioned it before. Not even the supermodel I used to date.
4 Fabrication	That wasn't snoring you heard, that was breathing. In fact, it might even have been *your* breathing. Have you considered that?
5 Reluctance	I snored? But it wasn't *that* bad, now was it? You'll get used to it. Everyone else has, including the supermodel I used to date.
6 Avoidance	I snored? That was a fabulous dinner tonight, wasn't it!
7 Righteousness	I can't believe you don't like my snoring. Everyone else, including the supermodel I used to date, found it soothing.
8 Acceptance	I snored? Sorry.
9 Ownership	I know snoring is a problem. I have UARS! What can you do about it?

By knowing what stage of denial a snorer is in, the snoree has a better chance of moving a snorer toward ownership of the problem. This may eventually lead to the search for a mutually satisfying cure. Be warned, however: These stages of denial do not progress linearly. For example, a snorer in Stage 7 Righteousness might move to Stage 4 Fabrication. In essence, a snorer will say just about anything to deny his responsibility.

To add to the snoree's frustration, even the last two hopeful stages are tainted with denial. In the breakthrough Stage 8 Acceptance, where the snorer actually admits he was snoring, he simply apologizes and moves on—like someone stepping on your toe in the street. The denial comes from what's *not* said—there is little effort to make any changes for the better. In Stage 9 Ownership, the snorer finally concedes there's a problem that needs to be fixed, but it's a problem that he didn't create—it happened to him like a disease or flimsy grocery bags that rip when you carry a carton of milk. Yet he still won't admit he needs to do something about it.

So what is a snoree to do? Even the most patient, understanding snorees will take one look at the nine stages of snoring denial and search for a faster way to raise a snorer's consciousness. (See Figure 3.)

Tape-Record the Infraction

The absolute quickest way to get a snorer to admit his nightly habit is to tape-record his snoring and play it back for him in

FIGURE 3

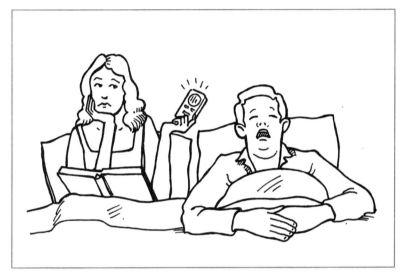

A Faster Way for Getting a Snorer to Admit Snoring

the morning. Better yet, play it back for him in the middle of the night. This not only gets the point across, it gets revenge. You may also want to tape the snore using an MP3 or digital device so you can threaten to either post his snore on a Web site or e-mail it to friends unless he seeks a cure.

Keep a Sleep Diary

A more patient snoree, or perhaps one looking for empathy or sympathy, might also keep a sleep diary as a way of proving the pain and suffering caused by a snoring partner. Here, too, while you might be tempted to smack the snorer with the diary instead of writing in it, confronting the snorer in the morning with incontrovertible evidence will certainly help your cause. (Please see Chapter 5 for a sample snoree's sleep diary.)

Take the Epworth Sleepiness Test at Home

The Epworth Sleepiness Test (invented in Australia) is a first measure of how sleepy a person is during the day, and hence a measure of the possibility that a person snores or lives with a snorer and is suffering from sleep deprivation. Score each activity for your doziness factor using the scale below and then total it all up.

0 = Would never doze

1 = Slight chance of dozing

2 = Moderate chance of dozing

3 = High chance of dozing

Activity	Score
Sitting	
Watching TV	

WHAT, ME SNORE?

Activity	Score
Sitting inactive in a public place (movie, meeting)	
As a passenger in a car for an hour (without break)	
Lying down to rest in the afternoon	
Sitting and talking to someone	
Sitting quietly after lunch without alcohol	
In a car, while stopped for a few minutes	
TOTAL SCORE	

If your total score is nine or above, chances are you're a sleep-deprived snorer or snoree—see a doctor or a marriage counselor.

If you fall asleep during any of the following activities, it is not an indication of anything wrong—it's normal—do not mistake it for apnea, snoring, or sleep deprivation.

Activity	Yes/No
Watching *Dr. Phil*	
Shaving	

continued

Activity	Yes/No
Listening to someone tell you about their dreams	
Going to any classical music concert	
Foreplay	
Listening when your father begins a story with "When I was your age . . ."	
Driving anywhere in New Jersey	
Reading anything about Kevin Costner	

Send Him to a Sleep Clinic

A snoree dedicated to quantifying the problem might also suggest that the snorer visit a sleep clinic to scientifically prove beyond the shadow of a snore its very existence.

Granted, a visit to a sleep clinic is typically recommended by a doctor in situations where a snorer's health may be at risk, i.e., the concern that snoring may be a symptom of something more dangerous such as sleep apneas or hypopneas. A visit to a sleep clinic can diagnose both the presence and severity of apneas. This will assist the physician to recommend an intervention such as corrective surgery or the nightly use of a breathing device (more on these cures later).

But even mild nonthreatening apneas or plain antisocial snoring and the loss of sleep to both snorer and snoree can be enough of a health hazard to warrant a visit to a sleep clinic. Please consult your physician as to whether you or your partner is a candidate for a sleep clinic.

My Visit to a Sleep Clinic

My doctor suggested I go to a sleep clinic because he was concerned about my drowsiness during the day—I would fall asleep in meetings, while reading to my daughter at night, and at stoplights. He felt that my snoring was a symptom of something else beside the fact that meetings are boring and so is reading about the Berenstain Bears for the fiftieth time or waiting for a light to turn green.

Going to a sleep clinic can be a dehumanizing experience. I arrived at 10 p.m. with my pillow and a book to read. This particular clinic was next to a hospital that specialized in sleep disorders. The two "sleep technicians" who greeted me had the lonely, dark-eyed, sleep-deprived disposition of late-night clerks at a 7-11 or vampires. Who else would take a job where you had to stay awake all night and watch somebody snore?

They ushered me into a tiny, medicinal-looking and Lysol-smelling room with a single twin bed in the center, and a column of blinking electronic devices by its side. After handing me one of those butt-freezing hospital gowns, they strapped nearly a dozen electrodes on strategic parts of my head, chest, and legs, each of which had a color-coded wire that plugged into the electronic devices. I felt like a lab rat or the son of Frankenstein.

FIGURE 4

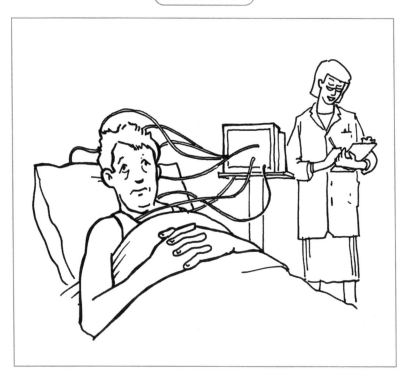

"Now, get some sleep!"

They told me to relax and get ready for sleep. Were they serious? They closed the door and went into the adjoining room where they could watch me through a dark one-way mirror and monitor my sleep data (heartbeat, brain waves, eye movements, breathing, and snoring) on their computer screens between checking their e-mail and playing cards.

I lay down on the hard bed and looked around. I was in a little white room that could have been a prison for Mr. Clean. The fluorescent light was brighter than the sun at noon, and I was wired for surround sound. I'll never fall asleep, I thought. Fortunately, I had had the foresight of staying up late the night before so I would arrive exhausted. I read for an hour or two and by 1:30 a.m., I actually fell asleep.

A few hours later, when I was deeply asleep, they came into my room and woke me for phase two of my test. They brought in another device that looked like an instrument of medieval torture. "What's that for?" I asked.

"This is a control," one of them explained. "We want to measure what your sleeping is like when your breathing is aided."

The device, known as a continuous positive airway pressure (CPAP) machine, looks like a fighter pilot's mask or scuba gear, or both. It covers only your nose, is held in place by straps that surround your head, and is linked by a long rubber hose to an air pump and a regulator. As you inhale while sleeping, the device pushes just enough air into your nose to prevent your soft palate and tongue from collapsing. Thus, no snoring and no apneas.

Nearly 3 million people around the United States sleep with this thing every night to stop snoring and sleep apneas. It is actually a life-saving device for them—a minor miracle. For me, it was a major inconvenience.

There is only one way to sleep with the CPAP device—on your back. So I tried to get comfortable and mercifully fell asleep.

Almost immediately, it seemed, my somber technicians, who now looked like exhausted vampires who had pulled an "all-nighter" (actually, vampires pull "all-dayers"), came back into the room to wake me. The test was over, and it was 6:30 in the morning. They ripped off the electrodes, taking thirty years of skin and hair with them, and told me to give their gown back (in other words, get dressed). Afterward, I went to the adjoining room and asked them to show me the results of my test.

"Did I snore?" I asked.

"Did you snore!" one of them replied with the sarcasm of a war correspondent who has seen it all. "On a scale of one to ten you were a nine," he said, and pointed to the needle-line chart that had tracked the decibel level of my snoring. "That's loud."

"You also had about thirty or forty mini-apneas during the night," he continued. "Which means you stopped breathing enough to wake you slightly but not enough to cause you any harm. We'll send the full report to your doctor."

Mini-apneas. That sounded cute and innocuously midwestern, like Minneapolis. Drunk from lack of sleep and delighted to learn that my snoring was legitimized by a diagnosis of mini-apneas, I returned home.

I would now be on a path to getting cured, or so I thought.

(**INSURANCE TRICK**)

If you are recommended to a sleep clinic and they find some disturbance, the subsequent surgeries or corrective actions (even if they're only to cure the antisocial snoring) may be covered by insurance. Otherwise, you're paying through the very nose you are trying to cure.

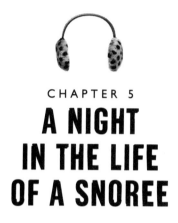

CHAPTER 5

A NIGHT
IN THE LIFE
OF A SNOREE

AS A WAY TO CONVINCE ME that my snoring was a problem—for both of us—my wife recounted for me all she went through in one night because of my snoring. I took the liberty of putting it into diary form. (Please note that her planning for, and anticipation of, a night of terror begins long before our heads even touch the pillows.)

4:00 p.m.   I am desperate for a good night's sleep. I went to the grocery store earlier this afternoon and got ingredients for a light salad for dinner. No steaks. No potatoes. No pasta. Nothing heavy tonight. Because when he eats like a hog he sounds like one.

6:00 p.m. Rob wants wine with dinner. I "forgot" to buy some. No wine tonight either because every time he drinks he snores.

7:30 p.m. He asks for seconds. Tonight, there are none. A hungry husband can get fat, even on salad. And a fat husband is a noisy one.

9:30 p.m. I have to get some sleep tonight. I tell Rob I need to get up early, so I'm going to bed early. I'll be fast asleep *before* he arrives and starts shifting gears without a clutch.

10:30 p.m. Tonight it's going to work. I know it is. I hope it is.

11:29 p.m. I'm awake! He's fast asleep snoring like a rhino. Why is he snoring? I did everything right! I nudge him gently. I cough politely. He stops for a few seconds, just enough time for me to think it worked. I try to fall back asleep. A few minutes later, it starts all over again. What a nightmare.

11:44 p.m. I'm still awake. He's still snoring, sleeping on his back. I move him onto his side. How come when people sleep they get heavier? I can hardly budge him. I'm married to a whale. A snoring whale. There! He's on his side. The snoring has stopped! Now I can fall back asleep.

12:39 a.m.   He's still snoring, and I'm awake again! It's after midnight. I hate him. No more gentle nudges. This time it's personal. I stick my elbow in his back. If I'm going to be awake, he should be awake, too. The elbow thing does not work. I pinch his nose, hard. Really hard. I surprise myself at how hard I pinch it, and how much I enjoy it. He gasps for breath for a few seconds, and I have a slight pang of guilt. Then he resumes snoring. So much for the guilt. I should have pinched harder.

12:44 a.m.   I can't believe all the sounds that can come out of a person. I prop myself on my elbow and watch with morbid fascination. I wonder, Is he drowning? Gargling? How do I write this out—ZZZGGGHHH? RRAAR-RRGGH? AKAKAKAKAK? Then there's the one that sends shivers down my spine—a gasping, suffocating sound like he's trying to catch his breath. Am I starting to feel sorry for him? Nahhhhh! I'm a woman without sleep!

12:56 a.m. If I were to fall asleep now, I could get five hours tonight, max. He's already had two and is headed for eight. Any way you do the math, it's not fair.

12:59 a.m. I watch the clock on our nightstand. I measure my life not in coffeespoons (sorry T. S. Eliot) but in digital blinks. 12:57. 12:58. 12:59. I start playing sleep games. Can I catch the instant the red dots change numbers? If I concentrate hard enough, can I slow the clock down? Oh my, it's one in the morning! No way am I going to get any sleep now. Tomorrow morning I'll look like a raccoon. I'll look like a *tired* raccoon. I will be cranky at work. I pound the bed with my feet. Guess what? He stirs and stops snoring! It's a miracle, so I seize the opportunity, and I snuggle into sleep.

2:05 a.m. I've had a brief dream of lying on a beach shattered by a horrible, horrible noise. . . . A motorboat engine? No, it's Rob!!!

2:10 a.m. It's now a fact, I'll never sleep again. Maybe I can stick a sock in his mouth. Or a towel. Or a sock *and* a towel. My friend once tried duct tape and almost killed her husband. I consider that an acceptable risk.

2:12 a.m.   I'll put a pillow over my head. No, I'll put a pillow over *his* head. Maybe a clothespin on his nose? A clamp? A jolt of electricity? What would Lorena Bobbitt do?

2:24 a.m.   Who's up at this hour? Just me and factory workers. I feel like crying. I question our relationship. I question my career. I question everything. What did I do to deserve this?

3:00 a.m.   I'm getting delirious. Time for earplugs. I tried earplugs once before, the industrial variety they use on airport runways, but they make me uncomfortable because I can hear my own thoughts. Rob gave them to me for Valentine's Day, can you believe it? These earplugs supposedly stop noise up to 34 decibels. Rob's snores have been clocked at over 80 decibels. That leaves 46 unaccountable decibels reveberating in our bed.

3:15 a.m.   Just as I'm about to put in the earplugs, he stops! It's a miracle. Maybe his uvula got tired. Wait a minute, he doesn't have a uvula. Maybe his tongue got tired.

3:30 a.m.   I don't trust the silence. I can't sleep. I know he'll start again soon. I close my eyes.

4:30 a.m.   I can hear the first chirping birds signaling morning. Can it be? Is that the newspaper slamming on the front porch? Please, please, please no. I need some sleep, just a little. I close my eyes again. . . .

6:00 a.m.   Beep. Beep. Beep. Beep. Beep. Beep. He set the alarm!

6:01 a.m.   Rob puts his hand on my shoulder. "Good morning, darling, did you sleep OK?" I am stunned he is so happy. Where has he been?

6:15 a.m.   I roll out of bed. I think to myself, What can I do tonight? I am desperate for a good night's sleep.

And it starts all over again.

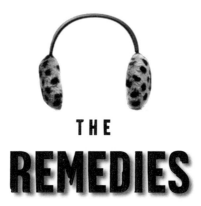

THE
REMEDIES

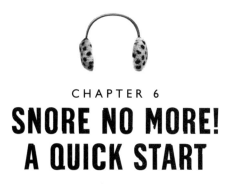

CHAPTER 6

SNORE NO MORE!
A QUICK START

BY NOW YOU'VE HEARD ENOUGH. Whether you're a snorer or a snoree, you want it cured. Most self-help books ask you to wade through chapters and chapters to get to the good stuff. Borrowing a page from software manuals, here's a "quick start" for snorers to snore no more.

Easy and Immediate Remedies

- Don't overeat at dinner.

- No snacks before bedtime.

- No alcohol two to three hours before bedtime.

- Avoid cold medicine or antihistamines.

- Avoid sedatives, muscle relaxers, sleeping pills, anti-depressants, or any mood-altering drugs.

- Sleep on your side, not your back.

- Raise the head of your bed slightly.

- Establish a regular sleep routine so that you do not go to bed overtired.

- Don't smoke at night.

Moderate Remedies That Take Effort (or Cash)

- Drop a few pounds.

- Exercise during the day.

- If your room is dry, get a humidifier.

- If you have allergies, reduce bedroom allergens (such as mold, pet hair, and dust) to reduce nasal stuffiness.

- Change pillows—get an orthopedic antisnoring pillow to keep your head and neck properly aligned.

- Get nose dilating strips or a clip to open your nostrils.

- Get chin strips to keep your mouth closed.

- Convince your snoree to buy and use earplugs.

Longer-Term and Expensive Remedies

- Stop smoking altogether (lifestyle change).

- Lose more than a few pounds and get to the average weight for your height and age (lifestyle change).

- Get a custom-fit oral appliance to improve your bite and hence your breathing (dental).

- Remove your tonsils (surgery).

- Fix your broken septum (surgery).

- Remove your uvula (surgery or laser).

- Reshape your soft palate (laser).

- Stiffen your upper airway soft tissue (radio frequency).

- Dilate your nostrils, permanently (acid).

- Sleep with a CPAP device (machinery).

- Sleep alone (human kindness).

- Sleep in another room or another country (travel).

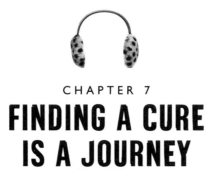

CHAPTER 7

FINDING A CURE IS A JOURNEY

WHILE YOU MAY BE TEMPTED to leap to the extreme remedies in this book, such as surgery or divorce, you should view this as a journey. Start with the easiest and least obtrusive remedies for both of you. If the simple remedies don't work, progress to the ones that require more intervention, more money, more commitment, and perhaps qualified medical assistance.

Curing snoring requires a lot of trial and error because there are so many reasons why you might be snoring. Are you a tongue-based snorer whose tongue falls to the back of the neck when you sleep? Are you a mouth-breather? Is your uvula enlarged? Are your nasal passages constricted? Are you allergic to something? Are you just too fat? Or are there multiple reasons why you snore?

Here are five simple tests you can take at home to help determine what kind of snorer you are and what cures might work best for you. First, make sure no one you care about is watching when you take these tests.

Nose Test

Look into a mirror and close one nostril with a finger. When you inhale through the other nostril, does the closed nostril collapse? If so, try holding it open with the eraser part of a pencil. If that makes your breathing easier, then one of the nasal dilating cures might work for you.

Mouth-Breathing Test

Open your mouth and try making a snoring sound. Now close your mouth and do the same thing. If you make a noise only with your mouth open, you may be a mouth-breather. In that case, a cure that promotes nose breathing (or keeps your mouth shut at night) may work for you.

Tongue Test

Relax your mouth and make a snoring sound. Now, stick your tongue out as far as it will go, holding it in place with your teeth. If the snoring goes away, you may be a tongue-based snorer, in which case any of the devices that reposition your tongue and jaw at night may work for you.

Uvula Test

Open your mouth wide in the mirror. Identify the uvula, that little boxing bag that hangs down in the back of your mouth. Stick your finger in your mouth (be careful not to gag) and gently place it under your uvula. Is it heavy? If so, you may have an overly large uvula and it may be appropriate to have it removed or reshaped.

Fat Test

Go to that same mirror again. Look at yourself. Are you fat? If the answer is yes, you may be a fat-based snorer. Don't lie about how fat you are. If you can pinch an inch at your waist, admit it, you are fat.

Remember, your destination in the journey to cure snoring is a solution that works for both the snorer and the snoree. And remember, too, the only thing more annoying than snorers are people who talk about life as a "journey." What they really mean by "journey" is that you'll probably never reach where you want to go anyway.

In this journey, there are remedies you shouldn't try at home. It goes without saying that only a qualified physician can assess if you need a medical intervention such as surgery.

Not that you couldn't rip out your own uvula or tonsils if you wanted to, but your insurance probably wouldn't pay for it. Moreover, if you see a snoree approaching you with a laser or a rusty knife, or worse, a rusty laser, ask for her health insurance co-pay before allowing her to operate. That should stop her in her tracks. There is nothing better for preventing wellness than the threat of health insurance.

Choose Your Doctor, Choose Your Cure

If you seek medical advice, be advised that the kind of doctor you see will determine the kinds of cures that are generally recommended.

General Practitioner. Will probably recommend you make lifestyle changes first: lose weight, stop smoking, sleep on your side. Will refer you to a specialist when these don't work.

Otolaryngologist. The specialist, also known as an ear, nose, and throat (ENT) doctor. Will also recommend lifestyle changes first, and then any number of medical solutions: nasal steroids, acid dilations, radio frequency shaping, laser surgeries, and CPAP machines.

Dentist. Many dentists are trained to help solve sleep disorders and snoring. Will recommend a custom-fit (meaning expensive) plastic device that positions the tongue and jaw to promote quiet, healthy breathing at night.

Sleep Physician/Sleep Clinic. Most major cities have a sleep lab or clinic associated with a hospital that specializes in sleep disorders. Will recommend a polysomnogram sleep study and other tests, and then any number of cures ranging from lifestyle changes to machinery and surgeries.

Marriage Counselor/Psychologist. Will recommend things like "owning the problem" and "talking through it" or "sleeping in different rooms" before recommending "cutting your losses" and "moving on."

Voodoo Priest. Will recommend buying a doll and sticking pins in it or creating a spell using a leftover body part.

Auto Mechanic. Will wonder why you are asking him about snoring. Mechanics typically put mufflers on cars, not people.

Please see Appendix I for a list of organizations whose Web sites can help you find a real doctor, dentist, or sleep clinic in your area. It's impossible to find a good auto mechanic, so don't even try.

61

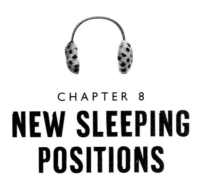

CHAPTER 8

NEW SLEEPING POSITIONS

Now that you have gotten your snoring partner to admit his culpability, it's time to do something about it. Hopefully, you've discovered that his snoring is not a symptom of something more serious such as a sleep apnea. Consequently, his antisocial snoring can be treated for what it really is—a pain in the bedroom.

The Snoring Sutra According to Rob

Like its 2,000-year-old cousin from India, which is perhaps one of the first self-help books ever written, my Snoring Sutra is a collection of sutras, or pithy doctrines, on how to improve your relationship in the bedroom and enhance your life. Only instead of focusing on sex, love, and devotion, it focuses on snoring, sleep, and lack thereof. Of course, it has some new positions to try—for sleeping quietly, that is.

Sutra Number One: Fall Asleep on the Quiet Side

They say all roads lead to Rome. Sleeping on your back creates multiple problems—all of which lead to snoring. Gravity and the position of your jaw team up to force your tongue and soft palate more toward the back of the mouth, restricting airflow that can lead to snoring. To make matters worse, to make up for the restricted airways, you breathe more forcefully, causing the already narrowed soft palate to warble even more like a loon. Finally, sleeping on your back also brings more blood to the nasal passageways, making them expand and constrict breathing even further.

That's why one of the easiest and fastest ways to stop snoring is to sleep on your side, positioning yourself like a Crescent Moon (also known as spooning) on the bed. (See Figure 5.)

Sutra Number Two: The Love Nudge

Going to bed with good intentions is one thing; remaining on your side throughout the night is another. A snoree quickly learns that as soon as her snoring partner unconsciously shifts

FIGURE 5

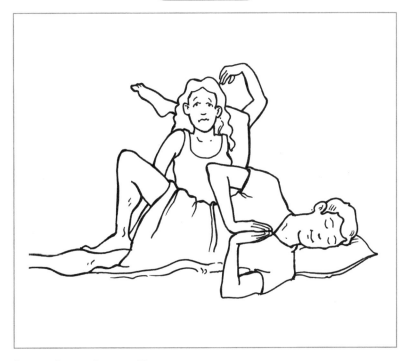

Snoring Sutra—Crescent Moon

to his back while sleeping, the trouble begins. When you see your snoring partner roll over onto his back, nudge, push, or use both legs and kick until he rolls over onto his side into the Crescent Moon. At first the snoree may approach the Love Nudge with some timidity, and you may even feel some remorse for disturbing your snoring partner's sleep. But as the night and your sleep wear thin, you will find yourself

with the opposite problem—restraining yourself from turn-
ing the Love Nudge into a hateful act of revenge.

The Love Nudge has another side benefit. In addition to
pushing the snorer into the proper sleeping position, it also
wakes him from his sleep cycle and disrupts the deepest,
most relaxed sleep—when snoring is its most profound.

(FACT)

A man went to a doctor complaining of mysterious chest
pains. After submitting himself to a battery of tests, he found
that his ribs had been bruised by his wife's nightly nudging to
stop him from snoring.

My wife has invented a very effective way of nudging
me. She has sharpened one of her toenails (although she
claims she hasn't, it feels like it's been sharpened to a
pinpoint) so when I roll onto my back, she can scrape the
sole of my foot, waking me instantaneously and prompting
me to roll back onto my side. Minimal effort on her part but
guaranteed results.

There are potential negative side effects to the Love
Nudge, especially when they become more insistent or
forceful as the sleepless night drags on. More often than not

the half-awakened snorer is either frightened by or resents the intrusion and might fight back with either anger or, in some cases, physical violence.

(FACT)

One woman who had been nudging her snoring husband—an ex-prizefighter—woke up to a right hook that the sleeping husband threw at an imaginary foe. Fortunately, he missed his wife but broke the headboard instead.

Sutra Number Three: The Gentle Prod

A safer way (for the snoree) to ensure that a snorer sleeps on his side is to use a device that "reminds" the snorer when he rolls onto his back.

(FACT)

In the Revolutionary War, soldiers would sew a small cannon-ball in the back of a snoring soldier's uniform to prevent him from sleeping on his back and snoring. Otherwise, the sound would either wake his fellow soldiers or alert the enemy. The snorers are coming, the snorers are coming!

In 1900, Leonidas E. Wilson of Broken Bow, Nebraska, received U.S. Patent No. 663,825 for a "shoulder brace and antisnoring attachment" (see Figure 6). This device consisted of adjustable, launderable, and ventilated straps that held a metal "prodding device" with four knobs or balls at the end. When worn at night, if the snorer rolled over onto his back, the prodding device would wake him and force him to roll over onto his side.

Since Mr. Wilson's patent, there have been numerous other devices that either prod, shock, or wake the snorer who rolls onto his back. For example, there is a sleep-sensing device that attaches to your back and beeps loudly when you roll over. You can also search the Internet for other similar devices.

If you don't want to buy such equipment, or don't happen to have cannonballs, another popular method is to sew a tennis ball into the back of his pajama top. It is often recommended that you take two or three tennis balls (or you could use golf balls or baseballs, but not basketballs) and put them in a sock and sew the sock to the pajamas. You can buy a pocket T-shirt, insert the ball, and have him wear it backward. Or you can even strap a pillow to his lower back with a belt. No matter what you choose, when the snorer rolls over, the ball(s) create discomfort, and he "learns" to sleep on his side. If you sew something sharp into his pajamas, the snorer learns not to trust you.

FIGURE 6

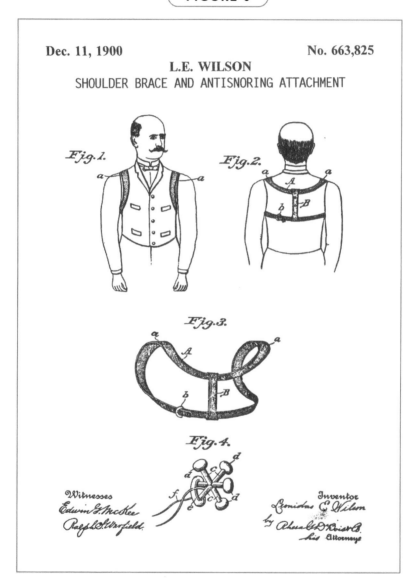

Shoulder Brace and Antisnoring Attachment (1900)

Sutra Number Four: The Perfect Pillow

For many snorers, changing a pillow can be the easy remedy that works. If your pillow is too fluffy, it may cause your head to be at an angle, restricting the neck and throat, and cause snoring. Other snorers have found that by *raising* their heads by sleeping on two pillows, placing a wedge underneath a pillow, or buying a special antisnoring foam pillow, they can open their airways without crimping their necks. There are pillows on the market that not only align the head properly to keep your nasal passages open, but also "encourage" the snorer to sleep on his side while cradling the jaw to prevent the mouth from falling open. If the pillow were any smarter, it would need a diploma. (See Figure 7.) There is even a patent for a pillow that electronically adjusts itself (and the snorer) for perfect alignments.

Sutra Number Five: The Elevated Bed

For some snorers, especially those who are overweight, elevating the entire upper half of the torso (not just the head with a pillow) works better to reduce snoring. If you do not have one of those luxury hospital beds with a remote control, place some bricks or a foam wedge under the head of the mattress. One sleep study in Australia found that snoring and sleep apneas were significantly reduced when the

FIGURE 7

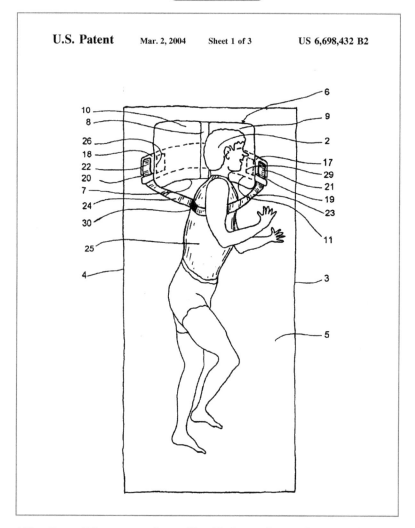

U.S. Patent   Mar. 2, 2004   Sheet 1 of 3   US 6,698,432 B2

A Very Smart Pillow, patented as a Movable Device Against Snoring in March 2004, has multiple foam components, straps, and belts to ensure the snorer sleeps on his side.

upper body was elevated by 30 degrees. Another study, also in Australia, found that people in a slightly sitting position at an angle of 60 degrees also had greatly reduced snoring. Finally, even though this was not studied in Australia, if the snorer stands at 90 degrees, he's probably not going to sleep and therefore won't snore.

When the Snoring Sutras Don't Work

For many people, all the positions, pillows, and tilts will do nothing to stem the tide. They will still snore. I tried all of my Snoring Sutras. I go to sleep on my side every night. When I roll over and start to snore, I am "nudged" back to my side. I have tried sleeping with tennis balls on my back, I bought expensive pillows, and I've tried sleeping on an incline. Nothing worked, and so in my journey to find a cure, I moved on to the next level of remedy—changing my lifestyle before I even got to the bedroom.

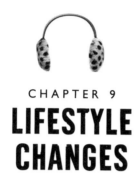

CHAPTER 9

LIFESTYLE CHANGES

EVERYTHING THAT IS FUN IN LIFE is bad for snoring. Eating, drinking, and skipping exercise routines in favor of watching TV are all lifestyle choices that affect when and how we sleep and snore.

By making improvements to your lifestyle, not only will you make your mother happy, you'll also improve your chances of stopping—or not even starting—to snore.

Establish a Better Sleep Cycle

Not only do we live in a snoring nation, we live in a sleep-deprived nation. Before Thomas A. Edison invented the lightbulb (and forever changed our waking and sleeping patterns by allowing us to have fun at night with the lights on), Americans averaged over ten hours of sleep each night, according to the National Sleep Foundation (NSF). Today, Americans average only 6.9 hours each weeknight and an extra thirty minutes on the weekend because we don't have to get up early to get a Starbucks from a slow barista on our way to work or school. This loss of sleep is why 70 million Americans report that they have some type of sleep problem ranging from snoring to narcolepsy to restless legs syndrome (where you run in your sleep like a cartoon character).

This sleep deprivation creates a vicious cycle among snorers and snorees. When a person who is prone to snoring goes to bed overtired, they tend to fall quickly into—and stay longer in—the "deep sleep" part of their sleep cycle. In this deep part of the cycle, the soft palate relaxes and the vicious snoring cycle starts.

Sleep deprivation leads to snoring. Snoring leads to sleep deprivation. Sleep deprivation leads to more snoring. More snoring leads to angry snorees who wake up the snorers out of revenge and this leads to more sleep deprivation and more snoring.

One wonders: How come we've never heard of a "kind cycle"? Why are they always vicious? It takes work to create a kind cycle; left to their own devices, cycles always turn vicious. The work I'm referring to is the restoration of a more normal sleep pattern so that you can get your minimum eight hours every night.

The National Sleep Foundation offers these tips for better sleep and minimizing your chances for snoring:

NSF Tips for Better Sleep

1. Maintain a regular daily and nightly schedule—including weekends.

2. Establish a regular, relaxing bedtime routine such as soaking in a hot bath or in a hot tub and then reading a book or listening to soothing music.

3. Create a sleep-conducive environment that is dark, quiet, comfortable, and cool.

4. Sleep on a comfortable mattress and pillows.

5. Use your bedroom only for sleep and sex. It is best to take work materials, computers, and televisions out of the sleeping environment. (You can use other rooms for sex. The NSF didn't tell me this; the *Kama-Sutra* did.)

6. Finish eating at least two to three hours before your regular bedtime.

7. Exercise regularly. It is best to complete your workout at least a few hours before bedtime.

8. Avoid caffeine (e.g., coffee, tea, soft drinks, chocolate) close to bedtime. It can keep you awake.

9. Avoid nicotine (e.g., cigarettes, tobacco products) close to bedtime. It can lead to poor sleep.

10. Avoid alcohol close to bedtime. It can lead to disrupted sleep later in the night.

As you can see, the very things that assist your ability to sleep—healthy eating, exercise, smoke-free living—also increase your defense against snoring. It's a compounding effect—in fact, it's the kind cycle I was just talking about. Let's take a closer look.

Lose Weight Now, Don't Ask Me How

The good news is, virtually all sleep experts agree that being overweight is the most common cause of snoring and, in many ways, the easiest to cure. The bad news is, if you haven't lost weight by now, can snoring—which is essentially the other person's problem anyway—be enough of an incentive to try? Perhaps if you knew what being overweight did to the *inside* of your neck, you might be inclined to diet.

Even a person who is ten pounds over his or her ideal body weight will have excess fat along all the insides of the throat. In other words, not only are you getting a belly, so is your throat. This constricts the airways, and as we know, *anything* that restricts airflow in your throat is likely to cause snoring. Moreover, not only is your throat getting fat, so are the *muscles* in your throat that control the soft tissues of your palate. As these muscles pork up, they lose some ability to control the soft tissues, increasing their floppiness and thus their tendency to snore.

If you are obese (which is now considered to be a national epidemic), then things really get bad. Not only is your throat constricted and your soft palate more floppy, but when you lie down—especially on your back—the fatty tissue from underneath your chin can roll back into your throat, collapsing it even more. At the same time, the extra weight from your belly pushes down on your diaphragm. This in turn makes your lungs smaller and further restricts airflow.

By the way, "overweight" is defined as being up to 20 percent over your ideal body weight. "Obese" means being more than 20 percent, and being "morbidly obese" means being more than 75 percent. There are many ways to calculate your ideal weight based on your age, height, and body frame, but one rule of thumb is that if you can pinch more than an inch at your waist, you're overweight.

There have been enough studies to unequivocally prove that losing weight works. Sleep studies in Finland, Denmark, Florida, Wisconsin, and Ohio found overwhelming evidence that when you lose weight the snoring (and the apneas) stop.

There's a healthy diet of diet books that offer advice on every which way to lose weight. Find the one that works for you and you'll reap many benefits.

Get Routine Exercise

Routine exercise not only helps you with establishing a better sleep cycle, it is mandatory with any weight-loss program. Here, too, find an exercise program that suits you and stick with it. Enough said.

Exercise Your Tongue and Jaw—Seriously

Some sleep researchers have experimented with an exercise routine that strengthens the jaw and tongue muscles to keep the mouth shut at night (and facilitate nose breathing instead of snore-inducing mouth breathing), and to help position the lower jaw and tongue forward in the mouth. The exercises include:

- Clenching a pencil or something similar (preferably not alive) between the teeth for at least ten minutes before going to bed or until the jaw muscles begin to ache. (See Figure 8.)

- Pushing two fingers against the chin while the jaw pushes back

- Chewing large amounts of gum before bedtime

FIGURE 8

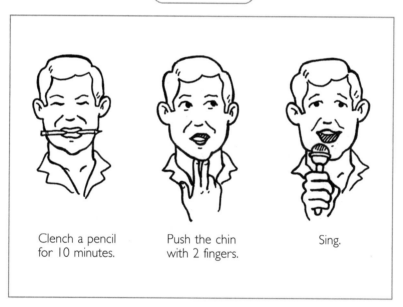

Clench a pencil
for 10 minutes.

Push the chin
with 2 fingers.

Sing.

Exercises to Curb Snoring

- Pushing the tongue against the lower teeth for up to four minutes

- Singing (more on this later)

While there is no scientific proof that this helps, the sight of your snoring partner doing tongue and jaw exercises is well worth the effort.

Stop Smoking

In 1988, Dr. John Bloom at the University of Arizona College of Medicine conducted a study on the effects of smoking on snoring. He found that women who smoked were four times as likely to snore as nonsmokers, and among men, smokers were two and a half times more likely to snore.

There are several ways that smoking increases your likelihood of snoring. First, the smoke itself irritates the entire length of the upper airways, causing them to narrow and lose muscle tone. As these soft tissues lose tone, they are more likely to flap when lying down and breathing (aka snoring). Second, nicotine increases your blood pressure and this narrows blood vessels and can affect the upper airways the same as the smoke. Finally, smoking tends to create insomnia (thanks to the nicotine again). This disruption of your sleep cycle can lead to increased snoring patterns as you fall into a deep sleep too fast and too often.

So in addition to causing cancer, heart disease, strokes, ulcers, shortness of breath, kidney disease, chronic bronchitis, emphysema, loss of sex drive, increase in allergies, infertility, birth defects, and wrinkled skin, smoking *also* causes snoring.

Need I say more?

Stop Drinking

How many times have you had a little nightcap before going to bed in an effort to get to sleep more easily? Little did you know that one drink before bedtime does just the opposite— it actually *impedes* your ability to get a good night's sleep. It also multiplies your chances of snoring.

Like smoking, drinking narrows the passageways in your throat—not by irritation, but by relaxation—and a narrowed throat is more likely to collapse during sleep and lead to snoring. Moreover, alcohol causes the blood vessels in your throat to engorge, again narrowing the passageways. Finally, alcohol disrupts the central nervous system and your sleep patterns, causing you to awaken several times during the night and fall back to sleep in a deeper, more snoring-prone way.

If you want to stop antisocial snoring, stop your social drinking two to three hours before bedtime. Everyone, including yourself, will sleep more easily.

Take a Shower or Buy a Humidifier

If you live in an arid or semiarid climate or you have hot air gas heat, chances are your bedroom is drier than an Englishman's wit. When you sleep, this dryness can lead to stuffed or irritated sinuses and nasal passageways, which, of course, leads to snoring. This also explains why Englishmen are stuffy and irritated when awake.

Buy a humidifier or take a long, hot shower before going to bed. But don't overcompensate. If you leave the humidifier on too long or take too long a shower, the extra moisture will condense on your walls and ceilings (as it did for me), and you'll find yourself in an unpleasant situation—an indoor rainstorm. The snoree will appreciate the silence but not the puddles.

Close the Medicine Cabinet

Any pills you take to alter your mood—muscle relaxers, painkillers, antidepressants—also affect your soft palate. When your throat is relaxed or no longer depressed, it gets so comfortable it starts to flop when you sleep. If you can, pass up the Prozac and do a good crossword puzzle instead. Even some (not all) antihistamines, which you think may help because they *open* the nasal passageways and prevent congestion, do just the opposite. While they're opening your sinuses, they are also irritating your soft palate and thereby creating an opportunity for snoring. In addition, some antihistamines such as those that use pseudoephedrine or ephedrine raise your blood pressure and cause havoc in your nasal passages. This disrupts sleep and can also lead to snoring.

While certain over-the-counter decongestants such as Afrin do provide temporary relief, most of them warn you about a rebound effect—if you use them more than three days in a row, you could actually end up more congested.

If you must take a decongestant at night for allergies or other reasons, work with your doctor to find one that does not also irritate your palate and cause snoring.

Get Rid of Allergens and Pet Dander

Allergies, even minor ones, can cause snoring because not only do they irritate your nasal passageways, they also force you to breathe more through your mouth. There are many, many ways to fight allergy-creating situations (pet hair, pet dander, dried pet slobber, molds, pollens, insects, parts of insects, and dust mites—yes, those little dust bugs really do exist):

- Vacuum your rugs frequently with a mold- and bacteria-catching filtered vacuum.

- Change the filter on your furnace or air conditioner frequently.

- Throw out old stuffed chairs, stuffed toys, stuffed pillows, stuffed sofas, and any hunting trophies or relatives you have stuffed in your bedroom.

- Wash and change your bedding frequently.

- Wash your hands often (especially after throwing out stuffed relatives).

- Have someone else do the housecleaning so you don't have to breathe all the stirred-up dust (this means you also don't have to clean the bathroom, which has nothing to do with snoring).

- During pollen season, sleep with your windows closed.

- In fact, when you stop and think about all the things that are outside in the air and inside in dust, you may want to stop breathing altogether, which also stops snoring in 95 percent of the male population (according to a study in Denmark).

- If your pet is a dog, ask it nicely to sleep in another room; if your pet is a cat or a monkey, lock your door; if your pet is a fish, it's not the problem, leave it alone.

When Pets Snore

Pets snore—mostly dogs, mostly fat dogs, mostly fat male dogs that smoke. Our dogs are getting fatter because we overfeed them with processed dog food, and they don't exercise very much, so they are snoring more.

Here's a case in point:

There once was a dog named Sumo, a mastiff who lived in an apartment building with his owner. The dog snored so loud that everyone in the apartment building heard it. The snoring set off the burglar alarm in one apartment, and in another, a couple tried twice to sue the dog owner. The dog was ultimately evicted for violating "noise pollution" ordinances.

---(**FACT**)---

Volker H. of Hanover, Germany, divorced his wife, Sabine, of eighteen years because her dog, a Labrador named Moritz, snored. As a puppy, Moritz slept at the foot of the bed, but as the dog got older he got louder, and Volker could barely sleep. The problem deepened when Sabine started feeding the dog dried pigs' ears in their bed, which made the dog snore (and smell) even worse. Volker gave Sabine an ultimatum—either the dog or he would leave. The dog stayed.

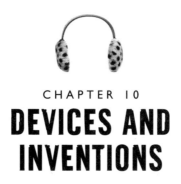

CHAPTER 10

DEVICES AND INVENTIONS

IF NECESSITY IS THE MOTHER OF INVENTION, lack of sleep is the mother of necessity (that makes it the grandmother of invention). Meanwhile, success has a thousand fathers. That makes antisnoring devices that fail the bastard children of necessity and bastard grandchildren of lack of sleep.

The quest for a good night's sleep has inspired thousands of inventors to develop antisnoring devices worthy of Leonardo da Vinci (or at least Rube Goldberg) for their inventiveness and arcane silliness. The search for the perfect antisnoring device that *finally* stops snoring, 100 percent guaranteed, every time, money back if you're not satisfied, is not unlike the quest for the 200-mile-per-gallon carburetor, the 20-year lightbulb, or the better mousetrap. Everyone thinks they have built a proverbial better mousetrap, and no one has succeeded—proverbially or otherwise.

In fact, since 1976 the United States Patent Office awarded 181 patents for *real* (not proverbial) better mouse-traps (see Figure 9). For example, "Improvements in Mousetraps," U.S. Patent No. 1,080,623, was awarded in 1913 to Jacob Brorby of Iowa and consisted of metal teeth that snapped shut over a baited mouse. Nearly ninety years later, "Rodent Trap with Entrapping Teeth" was awarded U.S. Patent No. 6,415,544 in 2002 to Rick Leyerle of Wisconsin and consisted of plastic teeth "closing against each other . . . thus striking and crushing rodents caught between the teeth, but minimizing damage to children or pets inadvertently actuating the trap." NOTE: Athough tempting, these mouse-traps should not be used as antisnoring devices on husbands.

During that same time frame (since 1976), the United States Patent Office awarded 791 patents for better anti-snoring devices—more than four times as many patents than were awarded for mousetraps. One can only conclude that snoring in the bedroom is more of a nuisance (by a factor of four) than rodents in the house, but a mouse that snored would still be a real nuisance.

In my personal quest to find a stop-snoring device that worked, I tried almost every kind of invention. I did not, however, show the mousetrap with teeth to my wife, since she

FIGURE 9

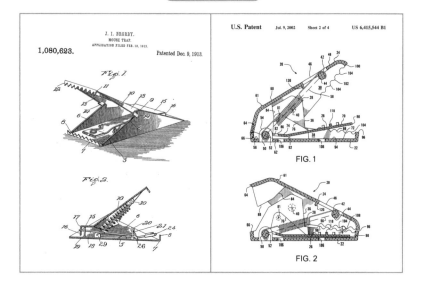

Better Mousetraps, Not Antisnoring Devices

would suggest this as an "acceptable solution" to my snoring on the theory that it takes a bigger rat to catch a mouse.

Antisnoring devices can be grouped by the particular kind of snoring problem they are trying to solve.

Nasal Dilators

If you snore because your nose or nasal passageways are the problem, i.e., they are too narrow or are easily congested, forcing you to breathe through your mouth when you sleep, then you should consider any one of the nasal dilator products on the market.

The most common and simplest nasal dilator is the *nasal strip*—the disposable drug- and prescription-free adhesive butterfly strip that is placed over the nose and lifts the nasal passages open. It is important that the nasal strip be placed properly or it will be ineffective (see Figure 10). It is also important that you remove the strip gently and carefully. When I removed my strip after a frustrating evening of snoring, I took part of my nose skin with it. Be patient: Strip manufacturers advise that it may take a week of usage before the strips have any impact on snoring.

FIGURE 10

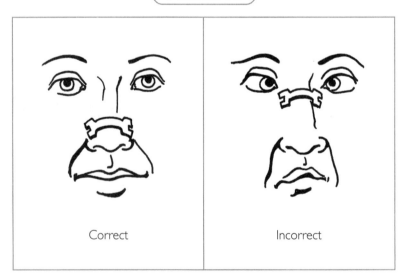

Correct   Incorrect

Correct and Incorrect Placement of Nasal Strip

They didn't work for me; I still snored.

There are several *nose clips* on the market that are inserted inside the nose and work to keep the nostrils and nasal passages open at night. Some clips keep the nose open physically—like a spring—either from outside or inside the nose. Other clips place internal pressure on the septum nerves: This stimulation reduces secretions and swelling while opening the nasal passageways. Other high-tech clips not only keep the nose open with a slight spring, but (because they have powerful magnetic chips) also stimulate the septum nerves, encouraging the nasal cavity to open. Here, too, patience and faith are required, since it takes three to five days and a belief in magnets before the benefits become obvious.

(FIGURE 11)

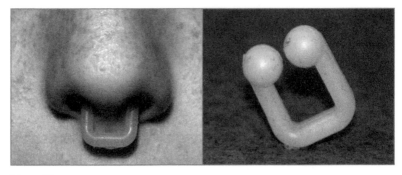

Nose Clip

All are reusable (after washing). But they didn't work for me; I still snored.

Anti-Mouth-Breathing Devices

Many sleep therapists claim that breathing through the mouth while sleeping is the most common cause for snoring, especially loud snoring. A study conducted at Rush University Medical Center in Chicago and presented to the Associated Professional Sleep Societies in 2004 concluded that proper nasal breathing dramatically reduces snoring and mild sleep apneas. Not only does mouth breathing force air over the tongue and soft palate, it also dries out the mouth—both of which lead to snoring.

Proper breathing is so important that many cultures have identified nose breathing as the essential link between health, mind, body, and spirit. Some Native Americans used to train their children to breathe through their noses while sleeping. Zen masters have always known the spiritual and meditative connection between breathing and spiritual health. Even self-help guru Deepak Chopra, MD, agrees: "Breathing is the link between the biological and spiritual elements of nature."

If you don't breathe through your nose naturally, then you may want to consider any one of the many devices that assist in this process. Remember that the sleeping pillows and postures I suggested earlier force you to sleep on your side and assist in keeping your mouth closed, while nasal dilators assist in keeping your nasal passages more open so you don't need your mouth to breathe.

One of the more popular and inexpensive devices to inhibit mouth breathing is the *chin strip*. Like its cousin, the nasal strip, the chin strip is a disposable drug- and prescription-free adhesive strip that is applied in a U shape underneath and around the lips. When placed properly, it keeps the mouth almost completely shut with the lower lip and jaw up, and the upper lip available for emergencies like coughing and sneezing. Your lips feel puckered and your speech is muffled; and, according to instructions, it becomes difficult to say "three gray geese grazing." (I had problems saying "three gray geese grazing" even without the strips.)

FIGURE 12

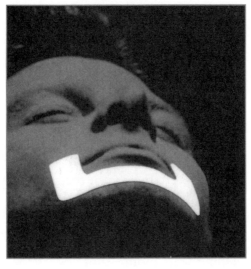

Chin Strips (Chin-Up Strips)

It took me several applications and painful lessons to get it right, i.e., don't put it on a sunburned chin. After about a week, my snoring did diminish. My wife was amused, since I looked like a raccoon and talked like a duck, and needless to say our sex life withered, as she is attracted neither to raccoons nor to ducks. Moreover, after I took the strip off in the morning, my lips and jowls remained puckered for about an hour, giving me the cheerful expression of a bemused weatherman all through breakfast.

After several weeks, however, my determined snoring figured out a way around the chin strips. I even tried pairing the chin strips with nasal strips.

It didn't work; I still snored.

(FACT)

A snoree almost suffocated her husband one night when she applied duct tape over his mouth to keep it shut; she hadn't noticed that he was so congested, he couldn't breathe through his nose.

Another popular device over the last century has been the *chin strap*—a harness of straps (either elastic nylon, Velcro, or leather) that go under and around your chin and over your head, keeping your mouth shut.

It's easy to see the inspiration for this device. When you watch an open-mouthed snorer, it makes logical sense to find a way to wire it shut. In 1900, Jacob Baughman of Iowa received U.S. Patent No. 649,896 for his "Head-Bandage" that forced the mouth shut during sleep without being "injurious to the human system" so that the nostrils, "the natural and proper channels" for breathing, could do their stuff instead of the "unnatural substitution" of the mouth. (See Figure 13.)

Gertrude Thomas received one of the first patents for this antisnoring chin device in 1909, for her "Chin Mask." Over the last 100 years there have been numerous applications of this device.

I tried one called the Snoring Stopper (once called the Sleep Angel and the Sleep Wizard), made of soft, washable stretch blue nylon. (See Figure 14.) This device also requires patience: The manufacturers recommend waiting fifteen to forty-five days to measure the effectiveness.

I tried wearing it for a month. I would yawn, and the strap would shut my mouth like a snap. I couldn't speak without sounding like Marlon Brando. I looked like Hannibal Lecter in *Silence of the Lambs,* bound tight so I wouldn't eat anybody. Every time I was amorous with my wife, she just laughed at me, and in the morning my teeth and jaw hurt as if someone had socked me on the chin.

And I still snored.

SNORE NO MORE!

FIGURE 13

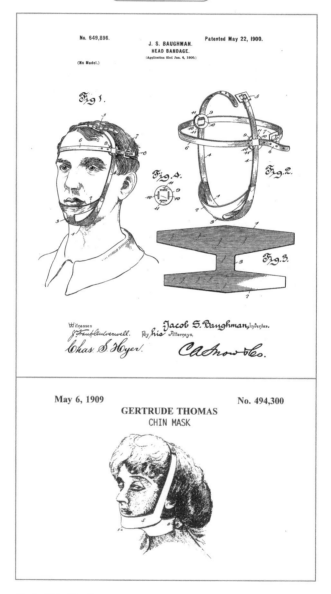

Early Chin Straps

FIGURE 14

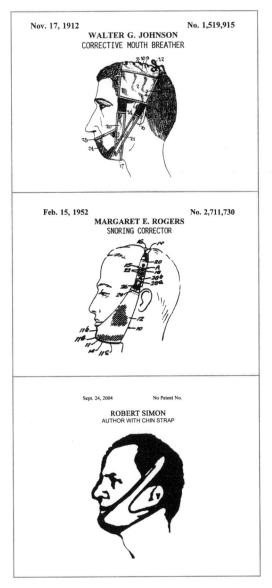

Chin Straps Through the Ages

There are other devices that also discourage mouth breathing. There are *mouthpieces* you can buy that attach to the outside of the mouth to prevent it from opening, and there are *neck collars* and *chin pillows* (see Figure 15) that surround and elevate your chin while sleeping. Make sure you get the right-sized collar as you do not want to choke the snorer—or maybe you do.

FIGURE 15

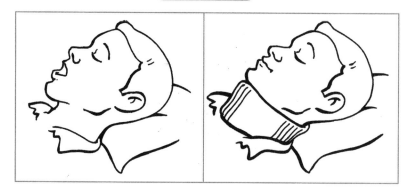

Neck Collar

FOLKLORE

There's an ancient folktale that if you cut a person's hair while he is sleeping and place a lock of it under a tree, he will stop snoring. Another folktale suggests you put an ax (unused!) under the pillow to stop snoring.

Oral Appliances

In this category, snoring cures require abbreviations because now *doctors* are involved. In the first year of medical school (in "Pricing 101"), doctors are taught the Hippocratic equation: The more complicated and official sounding the cure— the more you can charge.

That is why oral appliances are also known as oral medical devices (OMDs), because they are prescribed by doctors and dentists. OMDs can be broken down into two categories: tongue retaining devices (TRDs) and mandibular advancement appliances (MAAs)—all of which are designed to cure snoring. A TRD typically holds the tongue in a forward position so that it cannot collapse and fall backward during sleep and obstruct the airways to create snoring. An MAA repositions the lower jaw, or mandible, so it protrudes slightly during sleep and keeps the airways open. This device also works to (a) keep the mouth closed and promote nose breathing, (b) keep the tongue forward (since it's attached to the lower jaw), (c) keep the tongue more rigid during sleep because its muscles are constantly being stimulated, and (d) teach you to use the word "mandible" in a sentence.

There are more than forty different types of dentist-prescribed OMDs, most of them MAAs, and all of them custom-fit and expensive ($1,000 to $2,000).

Before you have a dentist or doctor prescribe one, you may want to try an over-the-counter oral appliance that typically can be purchased on the Internet for considerably less money ($50 to $200). Some are formfitting, and adjust to your bite using a "boil and bite" system where you get the plastic hot and then mold it to your jaw. Other suppliers will send you a mold so you can create a cast of your bite for semicustom fitting. Sears does not make oral appliances, by the way. They only make appliances for your home.

I tried a nonprescription oral appliance that I found and ordered over the Internet. I had received a spam e-mail about stopping snoring, and I was about to throw it out, when my eye caught a compelling offer: "Using high-tech impression materials, the consumer can now make a flawless impression of his own bite and buy a snoring control device for a fraction ($200) of what dentists charge for the same device."

When I called up to order, I also bought a teeth-whitening system (at a discount) using the same impression-making process. I was sold: Cure my snoring and yellow teeth all in the same phone call!

Within two weeks of ordering, my impression kit came. It looked very professional, and I was pleased—everything was neatly displayed in a box. To take my impressions, I had to mix a yellow and a white putty, mold them into a hot dog shape, and form it into the impression tray (first the top, then the bottom). Then, looking into a mirror (the instructions suggested asking a friend), I had to hurry and push the tray into my top teeth—since once the putties mix, they quickly turn to rubber. I held the tray in place for two minutes, salivating like a dog in front of a steak (a good reason why I didn't ask a friend to help). After two minutes, the putty had turned to hard rubber and my impression was made; I repeated the procedure for the bottom teeth and then mailed the casts in the self-addressed, stamped envelope. Easy.

Two weeks later my appliance came. (See Figure 16.) Molded in clear plastic, it looked like those fake wind-up teeth I used to have as a kid. It fit perfectly onto my teeth—hand in glove (or should I say tooth in mouth), and I was eager to take it for a test-run. The first night I wore it, I was concerned that it would push my lower jaw out too far, and I would start to look like a Cro-Magnon man.

FIGURE 16

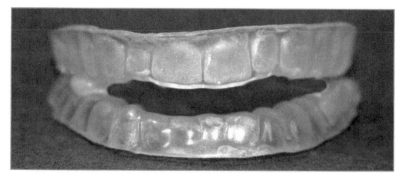

Oral Appliance

SNORE NO MORE!

I was reminded of my friend who had spent $2,000 for a similar device manufactured in England. I remember seeing her in profile at a cocktail party and wondering why she looked apelike. Later, I learned that she had worn her OMD so much, her lower jaw had actually started to shift outward. She said there had been some recent studies in Switzerland that showed that some users of these MAA OMDs were experiencing post-user mandible protrusion syndrome (PUMPS). I made up the syndrome and the acronym, but I'm not making up the fact that her jaw was really sticking out because she overused the device. Her husband was happier, because he preferred a quiet monkey to a noisy human.

But I was concerned. The first night I wore the device my snoring stopped, but I awoke several times during the evening with the startling sensation that I was choking—I had an overly dry mouth, and I was drooling excessively. Moreover, in the morning my teeth and jaw ached like I had been chewing on rubber all night—not a pretty set of side effects.

I decided to keep wearing the device because I thought my discomfort was modest compared to my wife's loss of sleep. Besides, the instructions said it would take patience— three to five days again—for the side effects to diminish and for me to get used to the device. A week later, they were right. The side effects, discomfort, and wake-ups were gone, and so was my snoring. In the morning, however, I noticed that my jaw was sticking out. Concerned that I was causing permanent damage to my bite and teeth, I called my dentist.

I learned that some morning protrusion was to be expected. My mandible muscles were tight from the repositioning at night, and that within an hour after waking they would relax and my jaw would snap back to normal. My dentist said I was not doing permanent damage; however, I felt compelled to do some more research.

According to two studies at the University of Sweden, there is only a small risk that using a mandibular advancement device (MAD), as they called it, will cause permanent orthodontic side effects, provided the device is made of soft rubber and does not protrude the jaw more than six millimeters. Nearly one-fourth of the 630 users in one study abandoned the device, and many of the others reported mild side effects (drooling, tooth shifting, and other jaw and mouth problems). I considered that an acceptable risk.

Perhaps that is why the FDA recently ruled that mouthpieces should be a prescription item only sold through dentists. Many online vendors believe this is collusion between dentists and the FDA and have gotten around the ruling by selling their oral appliances through European stores or by calling them "athletic" mouth guards. One Web site, which used to sell its oral appliance as an antisnoring device, now calls it a "sport mouthpiece" and encourages you to dream of playing football while you are sleeping (snore free, of course).

I wore my oral appliance for several weeks until, thanks to my overly powerful jaw and tendency toward teeth grinding (which this also supposedly stops), I broke it. There are two glued hinges on the back that keep the top and bottom together, and I ripped them apart. I called the company and they offered to replace it—or I could fix it with a glue gun. The other option would be to step up and get a more expensive and durable OMD prescribed by a dentist. But then again, if it is too strong, I'll end up looking like my monkey friend.

Back to the drawing board. I still snored.

Continuous Positive Airway Pressure (CPAP) Devices

Although I have never tried it at home—remember I did try it during my sleep test as a control—the continuous positive airway pressure (CPAP) device (see Figure 17a) is considered to be the one invention that absolutely works to stop snoring. This is different, however, from what you feel, look, and sound like while wearing it (see Figure 17b).

The CPAP (comprising a pump that sits by your bed, a flexible tube, and a mask that fits over your nose) forces just

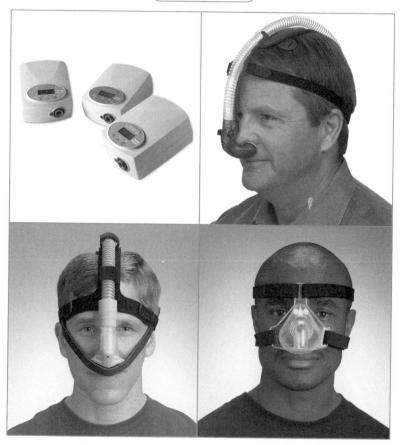

CPAP Pump and Masks

enough air into your nasal passageways to keep them open all night while you sleep.

There also is a bilevel positive airway pressure (BiPAP) device that is more adjustable and considerably more

FIGURE 17B

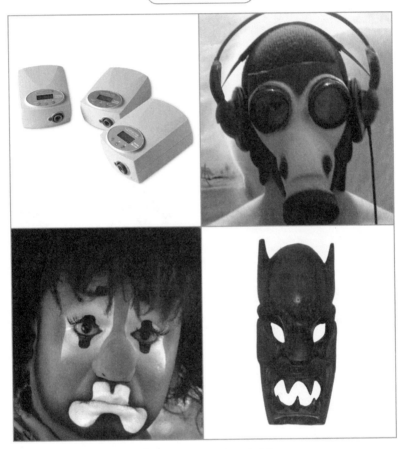

CPAP Pump and What It Feels, Looks, and Sounds Like

expensive than a CPAP. The BiPAP allows you to have different pressures for inhaling and exhaling.

While virtually 100 percent effective (users swear by it), the CPAP is expensive, ranging from $500 to $2,000 for a system depending upon electronic bells and whistles, portability, and mask style. That is why it is typically used by snorers with life- or health-threatening apneas. The good news is, CPAPs are typically prescribed by a doctor and your insurance company usually pays for them.

On the downside, they are cumbersome and may create some side effects such as abdominal bloating, dry facial skin, headaches, and sore eyes.

You also have to use it *every* night for the rest of your life, carry it with you when you travel, and unplug it when you want to have sex unless your sleeping partner is attracted to astronauts, fighter pilots, or Power Rangers, in which case you have bigger problems than snoring.

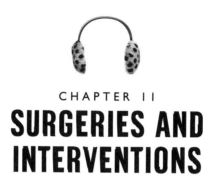

CHAPTER 11

SURGERIES AND INTERVENTIONS

IF YOU'VE TRIED EVERYTHING—new positions, pillows, nose strips, mouth devices—and you still snore, it's time to consider a more permanent solution. Remember, if finding a remedy is a journey, and both snorer and snoree are exhausted from traveling and getting nowhere, there are drastic measures you can take. It's possible to have a medical or surgical intervention that alters the shape and tenor of the snorer's mouth and nasal passages once and for all.

These surgeries typically are prescribed by a consensus of three people: (1) the snoree, the one who most wants the procedure done; (2) the insurance company, the people paying for it; and (3) the physician, the one who actually determines if it makes sense and then performs the work. You will note that the snorer typically has little to say in the matter.

When Children Snore

Children often can be some of the loudest snorers, creating gigantic sounds disproportionate to their size. When children snore, it is often the sign of something wrong that should be treated: enlarged adenoids or tonsils, or perhaps a foreign object stuck in the nose such as a piece of gum, candy, or rock. Moreover, approximately 7 percent of all children are born with some damage to the nose during birth—a defect that may cause snoring.

If the tonsils and adenoids are enlarged, a doctor will most likely recommend removing both (*tonsillectomy* and *adenoidectomy*), but waiting until the child is at least three years old. Nasal birth defects also can be treated with minor surgery. Rocks and other foreign objects (besides a finger) stuck inside the nose most likely will be removed immediately; the doctor will not wait until the child is three years old to remove the object—especially if the child is already six.

Seriously, children who snore may also have an apnea that can lead to dire consequences such as bed-wetting, fatigue, slowness, and poor performance in school (symptoms that may be misdiagnosed by parents and teachers as other emotional or physical problems). If your child snores, please consult with a doctor.

Minor Ectomies

As an adult, a snorer may have any number of physical problems in their nasal architecture that can be cured by minor surgeries. If your tonsils and adenoids were not removed when you were a child, and they are enlarged from chronic infection or just because they are—take them out. If you have tumors, polyps, or cysts in your nasal passages that narrow your breathing pipes, they can be easily removed (*polypectomy* and *cystectomy*). If you have weak nasal cartilage, which is typical in older people or those who have had cosmetic nose surgery (*rhinoplasty*), it may collapse when you breathe. *Nasal reconstruction* will take some excess cartilage from your ear or inner nose and sew it onto your nasal tip, strengthening it against collapsing, while giving you ugly ears. If you have *turbinate hypertrophy,* and don't even know where your turbinates are (they are above your nostrils, inside the nasal passages), and they are enlarged, you can have them reduced by either electric cautery, acid, or a laser. If you have a deviated septum because your nasal bone and cartilage obstruct the airways either from birthright or a broken nose later in life, this can be un-deviated (*nasal septoplasty*).

After I had tried all the lifestyle changes and mild devices to stop snoring and nothing worked, I decided to see a specialist. Following a thorough examination, my ENT doctor concluded that while I might be a good candidate for palate surgery, I definitely had a deviated septum—perhaps from some childhood trauma. I immediately remembered that when I was fourteen, Scotty Berman, instead of throwing the basketball to Mark Rotherman, who was waiting wide open under the basket, *wide open,* I said, Scotty threw it at my face, and it felt as if my nose had broken. Was that it, the birth of my snoring?

It didn't matter. The doctor said that before he did anything else he wanted to un-deviate my septum because one entire nostril was nearly closed by a misshapen bone and cartilage. He wondered how I could even breathe, especially when I lay my head down at night. Wow! So that's why I snore. I have a deviated septum. Suddenly my snoring sounded important. Although in high school I had always suspected that a deviated septum was a euphemism for a nose job. One by one, girl after girl would disappear for a few days and then return with this excuse: "I hab a debiated sebdum," she would say through her perfectly shaped but sorely stuffed nose. There were so many "debiated sebdums" running around my school I thought it was contagious. Perhaps I had caught it.

I was concerned. Would I, too, return not only snore free but with a new nose? I disliked my septum, but I liked my nose. My doctor reassured me, however, that the surgery only fixed bones on the inside—it absolutely would not affect any exterior look or shape of the nose. I was right about the euphemism.

The nasal septoplasty operation is actually quite invasive—similar to having your tonsils and adenoids removed. You must check into a hospital and go under general anesthesia. While the minor ectomies usually come with mild pain and discomfort, the nasal septoplasty (similar to adenoid and tonsil surgeries) hurts for quite a while afterward—like a severe sore throat that only ice cream, Mom, and painkillers can help.

After my operation, I had to stay at home for the weekend resting and recovering. My doctor warned me that my sinuses and nose would feel stuffed and pained, and that I wouldn't notice any significant improvements for a couple of weeks. Even with that warning, however, I was ill-prepared for how clogged my nose and breathing felt. Surely this was supposed to improve, not worsen, matters.

After the weekend, I returned to my doctor for his evaluation. He bent my head back slowly, peered into my nose, and then with a pair of tweezers pulled out—I'm not making this up—nearly three feet of rolled up, packed cotton gauze from *each* nostril. He was like one of those clowns who keeps pulling bananas, a string of hot dogs, or scarves out of his pocket—the gauze kept coming and coming and coming.

So that's why I couldn't breathe after the operation! No one had told me they'd be cleaning up my nose with two packs of rolled-up Bounty, the quicker picker-upper.

When he finished, I breathed like a man tasting fresh air after being imprisoned for twenty years. I was the Count of Monte Cristo—free at last. Everything looked great, the doctor said. My septum was un-deviated, my nose looked exactly the same on the outside, I was healing just fine, and in a couple of weeks, I'd stop snoring.

Little did I know that six months from that glorious moment I would be back in his office.

I could breathe, but I still snored.

A Brief History of Snoring Surgery

In the early 1960s, Takenosuke Ikematsu, a Japanese doctor, discovered that many of his patients who snored had larger than usual uvulas and soft palates. So, he did the usual thing that doctors do to cure problems—he began removing their uvulas and parts of their soft palates, and it worked. More than 80 percent of his patients reported that their snoring had been cured.

When Dr. Ikematsu published his findings in 1964, they were met by a fair degree of cynicism and disbelief from the medical community—the idea of *removing* a uvula and part of the soft palate seemed radical at best to solve a relatively minor snoring problem. Remember, at the time sleep apnea had not yet been "discovered" as a serious and potentially life-threatening illness. A year later, in 1965, teams of doctors in Germany and France simultaneously discovered and coined the term "sleep apnea."

One of the first surgical procedures developed in the late 1960s to cure sleep apnea and snoring was misguided. The *tracheostomy* cut a small hole in the trachea (or windpipe) just below the Adam's apple. During the day, the patient would wear a "plug" in the hole, and take it out at night for apnea- and snoring-free sleeping (see Figure 18). The theory was the hole would bypass all the noisy architecture in the nose and soft palate. It did, but it also bypassed all the *healthy* things nose breathing does for us like warming the air, filtering it

FIGURE 18

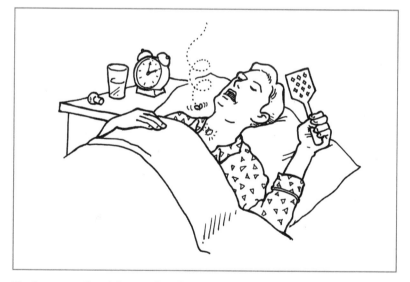

Tracheostomy Cured Snoring but Caused Other Problems

from germs, humidifying it before it enters the lungs, and keeping out flies. Aside from the fact that walking around with a plug in your neck like a tub-stopper was not an ideal way to live, the *tracheostomy* caused so many health problems and infections that it has been pretty much abandoned as a cure for snoring.

It wasn't until 1978, after numerous clinical studies, that the definitive work on sleep apnea, its prevalence among nonobese people, and its potentially life-threatening consequences was published. Consequently, sleep medicine and sleep laboratories began to evolve from a fringe clinical science to more of a mainstream specialty. In the early 1980s, a Japanese doctor in Detroit began to perfect the uvula and soft palate surgery pioneered by Dr. Ikematsu nearly twenty years earlier. Dr. Shiro Fujita's procedure removed the uvula, part of the soft palate, *and* the tonsils (if still there), plus some of the tissue in the back of the throat. This procedure removed a mouthful and became a mouthful to pronounce. The *uvulopalatopharyngoplasty*, or *UPPP* for short, was born.

The Main Event: Uvulopalatopharyngoplasty or Palatopharyngoplasty

Ever since Dr. Fujita's work in Michigan, the UPPP has become a preferred surgical treatment for chronic snoring and apnea. Initially, it was a three-day procedure, but now, it is typically performed as outpatient surgery under general anesthesia. You're in, under, and home all in the same day. Today, doctors report a 50 to 90 percent success rate in curing snoring from UPPP procedures.

The UPPP is not without its consequences, however. For one or two weeks after the operation, you will have pain—like a severe sore throat—some indigestion, and perhaps excessive drooling. There may be some bleeding, and in rare circumstances, some infection. For a very few, especially those who have a lot of tissue removed, the operation may cause some speech impediment. Others may experience discomfort in the back of the throat, as if something were lodged there that you can't cough loose. Since the tonsils (if you are having them removed as part of the UPPP) and the uvula play a role in filtering germs from your lungs, you may find that you catch more colds.

After my UPPP, my throat hurt like the worst sore or strep throat I ever had. I also drooled a lot. The good news was that since I could barely swallow, I also managed to drop a few pounds, which may have done more to stop my snoring than the UPPP itself. During my recovery, my wife also noticed that the operation gave my kisses the faint smell of burning rubber. I couldn't find a reason for that in any of my snoring resources, so I checked with my auto mechanic, who told me that when rotating tires, he sometimes noticed the faint smell of burning uvula. Go figure.

After the pain went away, I noticed another troublesome side effect. In addition to sweeping away germs, the uvula also acts as a windshield wiper of last resort, swiping away errant food and foreign objects before they get stuck in the back of your throat. Without my uvula, I found that a tiny crumb, a drop of water, or even some excess saliva (there's that drooling problem again) would cause an intense gag reflex as my throat struggled vainly to rid itself of the errant item. No matter how hard I tried, I could not clear the offending item.

It was a terrifying sight for my wife to watch a grown man suddenly and without warning start to gag and choke vehemently over nothing. The gagging was so intense that I was also speechless and couldn't tell her everything was OK; so I developed a sign language, wiggling one of my fingers left to right like a windshield wiper to let her know it was my missing uvula.

The good news is, after a few months, the gagging episodes diminished. Within a year, my throat had completely retrained itself to swipe away idle food and liquids without gagging. I don't miss my uvula anymore.

However, I still snored. I am one of those for whom the UPPP was not completely successful.

Laser Assisted Uvulopalatoplasty (LAUP)

A newer and less intrusive reshaping of the palate than the UPPP is the LAUP or *laser assisted uvulopalatoplasty,* invented by a French physician, Dr. Yves-Victor Kamami, in 1988. The LAUP removes less tissue than the UPPP. It does not remove the tonsils or tissue in the sides or back of the throat, aka the *pharynx.* The LAUP therefore is a well-suited procedure for antisocial snorers with only mild apneas.

LAUP differs from UPPP in other aspects as well. It is typically done in the doctor's office, not in the hospital, and only requires a local anesthetic—like getting a cavity filled. Because the laser procedures are done in stages, over three to five short visits resulting in gradual reduction of the tissues, the side effects, complications, bleeding, infections, and pain are kept to a minimum.

Doctors have reported that LAUP is effective in reducing or eliminating snoring and mild apneas in up to 85 percent of qualified patients.

(**INSURANCE FACT**)

Many health insurance companies will not cover LAUP, as they consider it "cosmetic" and not health-related. Check with your insurance company before proceeding.

A year after my UPPP surgery was not entirely success-ful, I returned to my ENT doctor in frustration. After all that pain, drooling, and retraining of my throat, I had expected to be fully cured. He suggested "topping off" the UPPP with some LAUP, using the laser to trim a little more tissue off my soft palate.

Indeed, the LAUP procedure was very similar to going to the dentist: show up on time, wait, read a three-year-old magazine about golf or travel, wait some more, sit in the operating chair with a blinding light, put on a drool bib, wait some more for the doctor, and then zap! A shot of anesthetic, a pass of the laser, and it's over.

I left the doctor's office exhilarated. This was the kind of high-tech cure I was waiting for. I couldn't wait to get home and go to sleep and give my improved palate a test-run. Of course, I'd have to wait a week or two for the irritation to subside to get a true test of the procedure. When a week passed, then two, then three, then months later and I still snored, I was depressed. I went back to the doctor asking him to "top off" some more tissue.

He was confounded. There was no more tissue to be taken off. My uvula, my tonsils, and my adenoids were gone—and my soft palate and my pharynx were trimmed.

What could possibly be next?

What's Next?

There are many surgeries that are used to correct apneas and snoring that I chose not to pursue.

Radio Frequency Reduction. This is a new procedure that uses high-frequency radio waves instead of a laser to reshape your palate. *Somnoplasty,* developed by Somnus Medical Technologies, was approved by the U.S. Food and Drug Administration in 1998. It cooks your excess tissues—like a microwave oven compressed into the size of a small pencil—to scar and reduce the bulk of the soft palate. It can even be used to reduce the size of your tongue, if that's the problem. Somnoplasty is similar to the LAUP in that it is minimally invasive, has mild side effects, and is performed by your doctor in his office. It is a relatively new procedure, and even though it appears to have success similar to LAUP, long-term studies are not yet available. Moreover, chances are your insurance won't cover it. Because there are few professionals trained in this new procedure, you may not even be able to have it done in your hometown. *Coblation* is another radio frequency procedure that is a rival to somnoplasty; it uses lower, cooler radio frequency waves.

Injection Snoreplasty or *Sclerotherapy.* Like somnoplasty, injection snoreplasty or sclerotherapy reduces your snoring by reducing or stiffening the upper palate. The doctor injects a chemical agent into your palate that scars, stiffens, and reduces the tissues. Relatively new, snoreplasty has met with mixed results. The majority of patients who have had it done say it works to reduce their snoring. However, some have complained that the results were short-term, and they suffered relapses, while others said it was a very painful procedure.

Cautery Assisted Palatial Stiffening Operation (CAPSO). Instead of using radio frequency waves, the doctor uses a probe that cauterizes and thereby stiffens and reduces the soft palate using electricity.

Palatial Inserts. Another new technique to stiffen the upper palate is the Pillar System, invented by Restore Medical, Inc., and approved by the FDA in late 2002. The Pillar System uses three tiny polyester splints that are inserted into the roof of your mouth—like the spines of a corset—to stiffen the soft palate and prevent it from snoring. (See Fiure 19.) Unlike a corset, however, these palate spines are not meant to come off.

Maxillofacial Surgery. This is a highly specialized surgery (only a few doctors are trained to do it) that either reduces

FIGURE 19

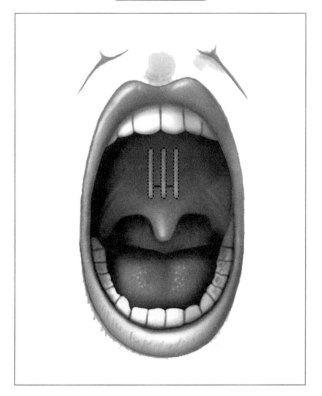

Pillar System of Palatial Inserts

the size of the tongue or reshapes the jaw to create more breathing room. And there are other highly intrusive *nasal reconstruction surgeries* that reshape the nose, nasal passages, and even the tongue for individuals with severe deformities that are inherited or acquired by trauma.

----------------------------(**FACT**)----------------------------

Surgery is not that bad when you consider the other alternatives. In 1923 a woman shot her husband to death when his snoring got to be too much. In 1987, a man from Winthrop, Massachusetts, strangled his hospital roommate (an elderly man) to death—for snoring.

CHAPTER 12

HOMEOPATHIC AND ALTERNATIVE CURES

FOR SOME SNORERS, after the surgeries, devices, oral appliances, and new lifestyle adjustments fail—and they still snore—homeopathic and alternative cures seem like the "natural" next step. For others, these holistic or new-age cures are the place to start—avoiding doctors, hospitals, insurance companies, and unnatural devices altogether.

(FACT)

In China they use an herbal potion of chives, alcohol, and wake-robin root to cure snoring.

125

Natural Decongestants

One of the most common homeopathic remedies for snoring is clearing your nasal passages before bedtime. Grandmothers have always recommended sipping some hot tea at bedtime to clear the head. Chewing honeycomb at night can keep the nose open, as can vinegar in water or citrus fruits high in vitamin C. One remedy recommends grinding a lemon or orange peel in the garbage disposal, and then leaning over the sink to breathe in the aroma.

One nutritionist has this homemade recipe to cure snoring: one cup of cinnamon tea containing two teaspoons of grated ginger, with honey and milk to taste. Or you can try one of the many herbal teas on the market that claim to open the nasal passages. These teas typically contain ephedra, the natural equivalent of the decongestant pseudoephedrine, and peppermint, another natural decongestant. There are also all-natural nose drops containing flower or herb extracts that lubricate and open the nasal passages.

Nasal Rinses

A surefire way to clear your nose before going to bed is to irrigate your sinuses with a warm-water saline rinse. There are kits on the market that include premeasured packets of salt and sodium bicarbonate, plus a bottle or sprayer that makes it easy (although unpleasant) to forcefully squirt the warm rinse up your nose. The rinse goes in one nostril and then out the other, carrying everything with it—and I do mean everything.

FIGURE 20

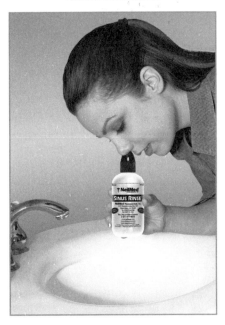

Using a Nasal Irrigation System

A friend who was a chronic snorer had used one of these nasal rinses and swore that it had cured her snoring almost overnight. Nasal irrigation sounded like something that would happen to a golf course, but I thought I would give it a try for myself. Here are a few tips I learned the hard way when irrigating your nose:

1. Use distilled water (either store-bought or by boiling water and letting it cool) so it's relatively germ free.

2. Warm the water before starting, as it makes the saline solution dissolve more easily, and it feels better than squirting a cold jolt up your nose.

3. Bend your head down over the sink and don't wear anything you mind getting wet.

4. As you squirt the water up your nose, be prepared for a sensation that is close to drowning.

5. Have tissues nearby, and do not allow anyone you know or love to watch.

I did this irrigation procedure for a couple of weeks and found some relief in the beginning. However, after gagging and feeling like I was drowning every night before bedtime, I still snored, so I abandoned the procedure.

Throat Sprays

Many people snore because when they breathe through their mouths, the air dries the backs of their throats, causing the tissues to be more flappable. There is an entire industry of throat sprays that claim to stop snoring either by coating and lubricating the back of the mouth or by slightly numbing and stiffening the soft palate. Many of them contain oils made from menthol, wintergreen, peppermint, anise, and cloves that both lubricate the throat and provide a decongesting or numbing vapor. There are even pills you can take now that release some of the same ingredients into your palate.

I tried a few of these sprays and while they were ineffective in stopping my snoring, they were very effective in making my breath smell like an herbal tea bag.

Behavior Modification

Some people believe that snoring is a learned behavior, and with the proper techniques it can be unlearned. Snorees subscribe to this theory, in part, when they pinch and prod a snorer at night, hoping that this negative reward will not only break his deep-sleep snoring cycle, but teach him to stop snoring. Unfortunately, most snorers don't remember the pinch because it happens during their deepest sleep, so there is no opportunity for learning. You could wake up a snorer first, and then when he is fully conscious, hit him, but that will only teach him not to trust you. More important, however, is the fact that a snoring soft palate is a *physical* reaction—it's not a behavior that can be learned or unlearned.

At most, a snorer can be taught through behavior modification to adopt certain sleeping postures that reduce snoring, i.e., sleeping on your side. The devices that zap the snorer when he lies on his back or create discomfort because there's a ball, wedge, or prod sticking into his back will ultimately teach anyone to change positions. Roll over on back—pain. Roll over on back—pinch. Roll over on back—shock. Sooner or later, the snorer will figure it out.

You could, of course, threaten the snorer every time he rolls onto his back, e.g., "If you sleep on your back again, I will detonate a nuclear weapon." After hearing this threat consistently over two to three weeks, the snorer will ultimately learn to associate nuclear explosions with sleeping on his back.

Some people have successfully used hypnosis to teach a snorer not to sleep on his back. You can buy self-hypnosis tapes and CDs that "teach your subconscious mind to help keep the right amount of muscle tone in your mouth and throat to allow you to breathe easily and quietly." Unfortunately, the same outfit that self-hypnotizes you to stop snoring also has CDs that self-hypnotize you to lose weight, achieve the ultimate orgasm, enlarge your penis or breasts, and grow hair. Imagine what would happen if you placed all of these CDs into a multidisc player and accidentally pressed shuffle.

My all-time favorite antisnoring device was patented in 1976 (No. 3,998,209) by Gilbert Macvaugh of Chevy Chase, Maryland. His "Snore Detector and Deconditioner" claims to use the teaching-learning procedures of Pavlovian and Skinnerian conditioning to break an individual of the snoring habit. (See Figure 21.)

Here's how it works: The snorer is first wired in multiple places to a machine that sits by the side of the bed, and he then theoretically goes to sleep. When an audible snore is heard by the machine's microphone, it wakens and *punishes* him with four "mild and harmless negative reinforcers." A bright light shines into his eyes, and a loud buzzer under his pillow rings in his ears. Then a cuff on his arm that's wired with a doorbell clapper smacks him, and finally a pair of electrodes on his other arm provide a mild shock.

To turn these punishments off, the snorer is required to wake up, change his sleeping position, and depress a switch for fifteen seconds or longer (to make sure he's really awake). At that point, the snorer is given two *positive* reinforcers—an M&M is popped into his mouth, and a tape-recorded voice says, "Good work." Now the snorer can relax and fall back to sleep, but if he snores again—watch out, the four negative reinforcers return.

Macvaugh believes that a snorer—as any snoree will attest—"soon forgets he was aroused by his own snoring noise

FIGURE 21

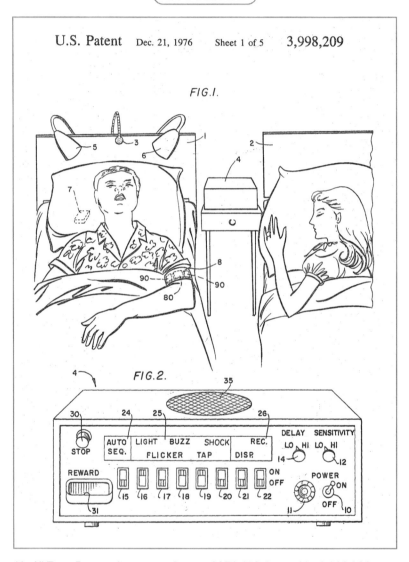

My All-Time Favorite Antisnoring Device, 1976, U.S. Patent No. 3,998,209, "Snore Detector and Deconditioner"

and starkly will deny that he was snoring." He continues, "Because of the lack of awareness of snoring, a snorer may realize in an *intellectual* way that he does snore, but usually does not believe in a *passionate* personal way, the magnitude and impact of his snoring on others." By waking the snorer with pain, the inventor hopes the snorer will now become passionately aware of his problem. Then by rewarding the snorer with treats, the inventor hopes the snorer will unlearn his acquired habit.

Upon hearing about this machine, my wife said, "Get me one of those!" She also wanted to know if she could adjust the electrical shocks. Unfortunately for her and fortunately for me, I haven't been able to find one in production.

Aromatherapy

Earlier I had suggested putting a humidifier in the bedroom to facilitate deep and easy breathing during sleep. Aromatherapists believe that herbs and spices can do the same thing. The practice of using marjoram to cure snoring comes from ancient Egypt. You can breathe more easily at night if you keep an open jar of marjoram oil by the bed, massage some of it on your chest, or place a few concentrated drops under your nose. Other aromatherapy oils use combinations of geranium, chamomile, and lavender, in addition to marjoram.

One aromatherapy for snoring uses oil derived from sea urchin shells from Australia. Have scientists finally isolated the ingredient that keeps Australian sea urchins from snoring?

FIGURE 22

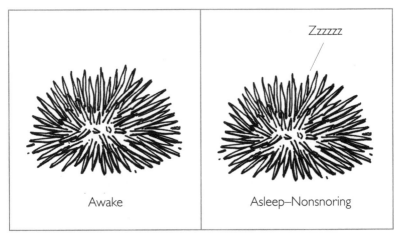

Awake | Asleep–Nonsnoring

Nonsnoring Australian Sea Urchin

Singing Therapy

A singing teacher at the University of Exeter in England discovered that "singing exercises can reduce snoring by toning lax muscles in the upper throat." The teacher, Alise Ojay, developed a series of singing exercises specifically designed to work different muscles of the soft palate, tongue, nasal passages, and throat where snoring occurs.

Given the choice between hearing you sing or snore, which would your partner choose?

Other Beyond-the-Fringe Cures

If you search on the Internet or open your spam e-mails, you will perhaps come across many other beyond-the-fringe cures. You can buy an exercise program just for snoring. You can learn to tone and strengthen your throat muscles (see Figure 23), and you can train your tongue to sleep in a better position in your mouth.

FIGURE 23

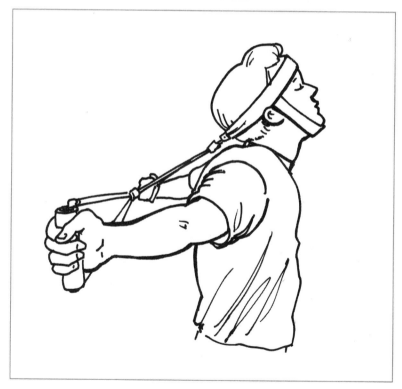

Exercising Your Throat Muscles

A speech and language pathologist, Janet Bennett, developed an all-natural exercise program that focuses on what she believes is the biggest obstacle to getting a good night's sleep—your tongue. She claims, "If your tongue doesn't know where to 'rest' in your mouth when you are sleeping, there's a good chance that it will partially block your airway, causing you to make undesirable noises, to sleep with your mouth open, or to gasp and choke for air." A series of simple exercises teaches your tongue to rest in a position that helps you breathe and sleep better.

If you don't feel like exercising your tongue at night after a hard day of using it for eating and speaking, you can wear a therapeutic ring that rechannels your snoring energy by using acupressure. (See Figure 24.) Wear the silver ring on the small finger of your left hand, and the ring's small pressure points send throat-healing messages to your brain.

You can buy an ionizer that pumps negative ions (like the kind created by a waterfall) into your bedroom. You can also wear an antisnoring bracelet that detects when you snore and then sends small electrical impulses into your wrist so that you learn to sleep on your side.

FIGURE 24

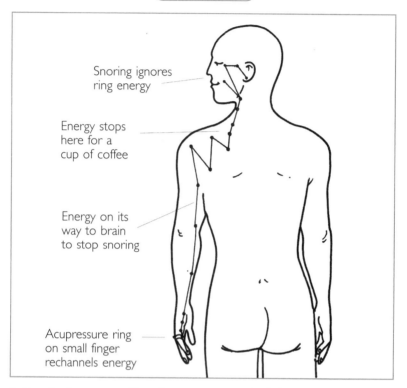

Snoring ignores ring energy

Energy stops here for a cup of coffee

Energy on its way to brain to stop snoring

Acupressure ring on small finger rechannels energy

Antisnoring Acupressure Ring places pressure on the little finger of the left hand, which allows energy to flow through body to brain to cure snoring

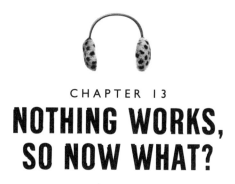

CHAPTER 13

NOTHING WORKS, SO NOW WHAT?

BY NOW, YOU'RE AT THE END OF YOUR ROPE. You've tried everything, and you still snore. The snoree is at the end of her rope, too. In fact, if she had a rope, she would probably hang you with it, then take your rope and tie your mouth shut.

The Mayo Clinic's sleep disorder clinic actually has a term for this feeling: "spousal arousal syndrome." It occurs when a snoree's sleep is repeatedly interrupted by a snorer. The snoree then begins to demonstrate apnea-like symptoms. She is irritable. She gets headaches. She has memory loss. Her sex drive is diminished. She is prone to accidents. She shouldn't operate heavy machinery. She shouldn't operate light machinery, either. Her mother thinks she should take a job that doesn't have any machinery at all. She has homicidal thoughts.

Another study quantified that a snoree might lose up to one hour of sleep per night from these frequent interruptions from the snorer. When you do the math, that's enough lost sleep to make anyone crazy.

(FACT)

According to one survey of nearly 5,000 snoring couples, about 80 percent end up in separate bedrooms during the night.

It's time for the snoree to take things into her own hands or put things into her ears to get through the night.

Earplugs

Earplugs are rated by their ability to cancel out sound under a noise reduction rating (NRR) system. Most earplugs, including the ones worn by mechanics at airports, have an NRR rating of between twenty-two and thirty and are made of either rolled and waxed cotton, pure wax, moldable foam, or silicone. The absolute highest rating for a foam, wax, silicone, or moldable plug is NRR-33, and it's made of premolded silicone rubber filled with a silicone gel for a perfectly tight fit. At NRR-33, a vacuum cleaner of 75 decibels is reduced to the sound of a whisper.

FIGURE 25

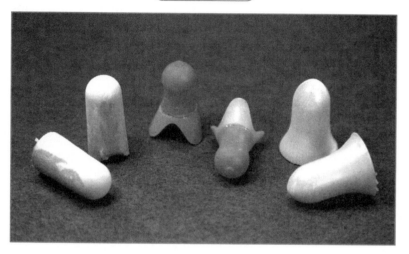

A Selection of Earplugs

LATE-BREAKING NEWS

A Taiwan company just introduced a "next-generation" earplug that it claims will be the highest-rated noise-reducing plug on the market, quieting sounds up to 37 decibels.

However, since more than 85 percent of snoring is louder than 38 decibels, even the next-generation earplug described above won't be enough. You can also buy sound-canceling *earmuffs:* When you combine these with earplugs, they will cut the sound out even further.

(**FACT**)

A woman in California slept through an earthquake of 6.9 on the Richter scale because it was quieter than her husband's snoring, which was more than 50 decibels.

The fit is more important than the Richter scale, decibel level, or NRR rating. A plug with a higher rating that doesn't fit in your ear is less effective than a lower-rated plug that is snug. Earplugs are cheap, and I recommend buying several different kinds until you find one that fits well and is comfortable to wear. You can even buy variety packs that have all kinds of different plug samples to test your preference.

(**FACT**)

Even when your ear canals are completely blocked with earplugs, you can still "hear" sounds through the bones in your jaw and head that lead to your inner ear.

White Noise

If you can't get rid of the snoring noise, you can always cover it up. White noise is the process by which the irritating rasping sound of snoring is masked to the snoree—in effect drowned out—by a continuous and soothing sound, like that of a rainstorm, surf, or a waterfall. You can buy white noise machines with several levels and varieties of white noise. The machines can sit by your bedside or hang from the ceiling, and they come with batteries and travel packs. The advantage of a white noise machine is that it plays continuous sound throughout the night; the disadvantage is that they tend to have a limited variety of sounds from which to choose.

There also are pink noise machines. Pink noise is white noise that has been filtered and altered to impact lower-frequency sounds and may be better suited to mask the rumbling of snoring.

If you want something less expensive with more choice, you can use a white or pink noise CD that you play on automatic repeat. However, when the hour-long CD restarts, those few seconds may be just enough to wake you up.

The sine qua non of white noise CDs is a CD that is created to mask out the specific snoring sounds in your bedroom. For a pricey $250, you can send a tape of the snoring to the white noise technician, who then mixes sounds designed to mask your partner's snoring. Make sure white noise works, and that you are planning to stay with your partner, before you try this expensive route.

The pinnacle of white noise machines is a device that completely eliminates up to 80 decibels of sound. Shaped like a hearing aid and using similar technology, the battery-operated device fits snugly into both ears and emits a total noise-blocking white noise. Be warned: The device is so good it also blocks out sounds you may want to hear like smoke alarms, crying babies, and late-night phone calls from your mother.

The Etiquette of Separate Rooms

If the survey is correct that in nearly 80 percent of couples someone sleeps in another room—the question is, who leaves? Although the snoree is typically the one to discover the problem, why should she be the one to leave the room? The late-night discussions and arguments as to whose turn it is to sleep on the couch, join the kids, visit the dog, or sleep in the bathroom can be as destructive and hurtful as the lost sleep itself.

FACT

On one of the snoring Web sites, a woman confessed that she had fixed up her marble bathtub with pillows and blankets so she could sleep there when her husband snored.

FACT

During one of our vacations, I was snoring so badly, I slept in our hotel room's bathtub. It was not marble, and I didn't have enough pillows or blankets, but I did save the vacation and our relationship.

Breaking Up

Unfortunately, the ultimate solution to snoring may be breaking up, and, in fact, snoring has been cited as grounds for divorce in numerous cases around the country.

---(**FACT**)---

Sarah Wilson will lose her third husband because of her snoring. On a divorce support Web site (www.divorcemagazine.com), the former nurse from the United Kingdom confessed, "I can see things with Steve going the same way as they did with my first two husbands. They both loved me, but neither of them could stand my snoring." After two and a half years of marriage, "Steve started looking tired in the mornings. He wasn't getting any sleep, and I thought, 'Oh no, not again.'" Steve said, "Sarah's snoring has put us through hell." He had to quit his job as a telecom worker because he would fall asleep on his ladder while fixing cables. Her ex-husbands have called her Darth Vader because of the grunts she makes— she is so loud, her snoring can penetrate walls.

In fact, snoring may be the reason you're not together with someone in the first place. Most snoring books and resources say that if your girlfriend refuses to marry you, it may be a sign that you are snoring. It also may be a sign you're a jerk. I would recommend a controlled experiment.

Next time you propose, do it this way: "If I stopped snoring, will you marry me?" If she says yes, buy her an engagement ring and some earplugs. If she says no, find another girlfriend.

CHAPTER 14

REVENGE: FINALLY, YOU, TOO, CAN SNORE

(Five Steps in Just Six Weeks)

BECAUSE MOST SNORING CURES are like putting a girdle on a fat man—the bulges always come out someplace else— perhaps there really isn't a cure. In that case, the only thing you can do is to get revenge: Learn to snore yourself. Here are five easy steps you can take to become one of the 90 million snorers who torture their partners. I guarantee sound results and revenge in just six weeks.

1. *Gain three to five pounds.*

    If you don't snore, it's because your soft palate doesn't have enough tissue to make noise. So, how do you get the extra tissue? It's easy—get fat. When you overeat, your face, neck, tongue, and palate get fat, too.

There are side benefits to this approach: the fun of gaining weight and the look of horror on your partner's face when you not only snore like Jesse Ventura, you look like him, too.

2. *Smoke and drink before bedtime.*

Anything that interferes with those same soft palate tissues will increase your chances of snoring. Smoking and antihistamines, which irritate the palate, and alcohol, which relaxes the palate, do it the best.

Imagine your partner's surprise when, after you have finished a 5,000-calorie meal (to get fat, remember), you stumble into bed to enjoy a smoke, a cocktail, and a NyQuil—all while lying proudly on your back. You should be snoring like a rhino; and even if you're not, at the very least, your partner will be very annoyed.

3. *Grow your uvula and tongue.*

If you have a skinny, normal uvula or tongue, you probably won't snore. This means you have no choice but to grow them. This takes practice and exercise—fifteen minutes, three times every day. Move your tongue twenty times to the right, twenty to the left, then up, down, into the back of your throat, and then out. Now do the same with your uvula—right, left, up, down, in, and out. I guarantee that in three weeks your tongue and uvula will be enlarged and you'll be snoring; if not, invite your partner to watch. Either way, he won't want to sleep with you.

4. *Use a start-snoring device.*

You can try enlarging your tonsils or adenoids through hypnosis. You can have silicone implants placed in your nasal passages or stick beans up your nose to constrict your breathing. You can wear a tongue enlarging device (TED) or a mandibular promoting device (MPD) that closes the back of your throat to promote snoring. You can wear a clothespin on your nose to foster mouth breathing. You can buy homeopathic sprays that irritate your throat with the essence of cactus, caffeine, and tree bark. You can irrigate your nose with vinegar or gargle with tacks. Or you can buy the continuous vacuum airway pressure (CVAP) machine, which fits on your face like a pilot's mask and sucks air from your throat, forcing you to gag and snore.

5. *Try microchipplasty (MCP).*

If all else fails and you still don't snore, there is an experimental procedure known as *microchipplasty*

(MCP) that installs a sound-producing microchip in your larynx. Pioneered by a sound lab in Sweden, MCP has proven to be effective in 98 percent of its clinical trials. The chip is activated by the REM cycle when you sleep and mimics snoring by stimulating your pharynx with one of ten prerecorded snores, randomly selected throughout the night at varying decibel levels. You can even have celebrity snores programmed. Orson Welles and the Three Stooges have been the most popular to date. Pick your snores. Set your decibel levels. Dial up your frequency. You're snoring now.

If these five steps fail, then visit the Web site www.startsnoring.com for a complete list of ways to start snoring.

Of course, none of these devices nor this Web site exist, but they should. Revenge would be sweet.

"Finally, a cure for snoring that really works."

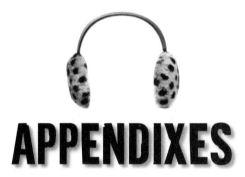

APPENDIXES

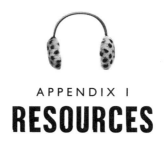

RESOURCES

Organizations

- *Academy of Dental Sleep Medicine.* Professional society of dentists who specialize in oral surgery and dental appliances to cure snoring, apneas, and other sleep disorders. Use "Find a Dentist" to locate a sleep medicine dentist in your area. www.dentalsleepmed.org

- *American Academy of Otolaryngology—Head and Neck Surgery.* Professional organization for ear, nose, and throat doctors. Use "Find an Otolaryngologist" for an ENT doctor (snoring and apnea specialist) near you. www.entnet.org

- *American Academy of Sleep Medicine.* Professional organization of scientists, clinicians, and physicians involved in sleep medicine and research. Use "Find a Sleep Center" to find a sleep clinic in your area. www.aasmnet.org

- *American Sleep Apnea Association.* Nonprofit organization with support groups (A.W.A.K.E.), resources, information, and links. www.sleepapnea.org

- *British Snoring and Sleep Apnoea Association.* A commercial organization for the 15 million snorers and their snoree partners in the United Kingdom. The Web site has well-organized information, resources, and links. It also has a snoring "shop" for online products and cures. www.britishsnoring.co.uk

- *National Institutes of Health.* The NIH, as part of the U.S. Department of Health and Human Services, is the national gatekeeper for medical research. Provides detailed information and articles on snoring, sleep disorders, and apneas through their online library, MedlinePLUS. www.nih.gov

- *National Sleep Foundation (NSF).* An independent nonprofit organization dedicated to understanding sleep and sleep disorders. www.sleepfoundation.org

Information Web Sites

- *www.mayoclinic.com.* One of the leading health-care centers; also has a Web site to provide information on snoring, apneas, and sleep disorders.

- *www.putanendtosnoring.com.* An excellent site even though it is sponsored by a commercial company specializing in antisnoring products (palate inserts and a mouth guard).

- *www.sleepdentist.ca.* A Web site by a dentist specializing in sleep disorders, snoring, and apneas. It has a very good overview of snoring and provides useful information on oral appliances used to cure it.

- *www.sleepnet.com.* A good portal that links to all things having to do with sleep and sleep disorders with information, links, and public forums.

- *www.WebMD.com.* A good introduction to snoring basics, symptoms, and remedies. Search "snoring" and choose your topics.

Books

- *Don't Snore Anymore: Your Complete Guide to a Quiet Night's Sleep,* by Jeffrey N. Hausfeld, MD

- *No More Snoring: A Proven Program for Conquering Snoring and Sleep Apnea,* by Victor Hoffstein, MD, and Shirley Linde, PhD

- *Restless Nights: Understanding Snoring and Sleep Apnea,* by Peretz Lavie

- *Sleep Apnea: The Phantom of the Night,* by T. Scott Johnson, MD, William A. Broughton, MD, and Jerry Halberstadt

- *Snoring and Sleep Apnea: Sleep Well, Feel Better,* by Ralph A. Pascualy, MD, and Sally Warren Soest

- *The Snoring Cure: Simple Steps to Getting a Good Night's Sleep,* by Laurence A. Smolley, MD, and Debra Fulghum Bruce

- *Snoring from A to ZZZZ: Proven Cures for the Night's Worst Nuisance,* by Derek S. Lipman, MD

- *Wake Up! You're Snoring . . . : A Guide to Diagnosis and Treatment,* by David O. Volpi, MD, and Josh L. Werber, MD

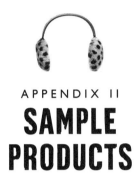

SAMPLE PRODUCTS

THE FOLLOWING LISTS of antisnore products can be found on the Internet or at your local pharmacy. Many of these products are listed and linked on the excellent Web site www.putanendtosnoring.com. (NOTE: You will also find list(s) devoted to new surgical procedures, and alternative cures, and one for snorees only.)

The lists are by no means an endorsement of these products. In fact, there is no guarantee that the names of the products are still the same (an antisnoring product may resurface under another name after a few years of disappointing users)—or that the products are even still available. Nor is any list comprehensive. With nearly 800 U.S. patents for antisnoring products since 1976, I'm sure I missed a few.

NOTE: According to urban legend, if you see a pair of sneakers hanging from a telephone or electrical wire, it means there's an antisnoring dealer somewhere in the vicinity. Please, do not buy your antisnoring products from street dealers or from Canada, as there is no guarantee you are getting the real thing. Ask your doctor, pharmacist, or favorite search engine for a reputable product, store, or online merchant.

SAMPLE PRODUCTS

Pillows and Sleep Posture Devices

Name	Description	Web Site	Avg. $
Comfort Direct	Variety of self-adjusting and mechanical mattresses and beds	mattresses-beds.com	Up to $1,000s
Dr. Parker's Snore Relief Cushion	Pillow straps to your back so you sleep on your side; includes video and booklet	endsnoringnow.com	$80
Dux Bed	Several posture-correcting mattresses and adjustable beds; also allergy-proof linens	duxbed.com	Up to $1,000s
Head-to-Side-Roller Pillow	Inflatable pillow forces head to sleep on its side	snoringcure.ca/anti_snoring_pillow.htm	$60
Lands' End Back-Sleep Pillow	Downlike filling supports neck for back sleepers	sears.com	$40
Makura Miracle Pillow	All-natural buckwheat promotes good sleep posture	makura.com	$45

continued

Pillows and Sleep Posture Devices (*Continued*)

Name	Description	Web Site	Avg. $
No-Snore Pillow	Foam pillow keeps your passageways open whether you're on your side or back	backbraces.com	$25
Original Silent Nightshirt	White nightshirt with foam insert on back	silent-night.com/nightshirt.html	$35
PAPillow	For CPAP users who sleep on side or stomach	sleepestore.com/pillows.html	$60
Sealy Posturepedic Snore Reduction Pillow	"Memory foam" promotes good posture	Most sleep and e-retailers	$50
Thera-P Antisnoring Cradle Pillow	Foam and bar construction keep sleeper on side	snoringshop.com/pillow.htm	$50

SAMPLE PRODUCTS

Nasal Strips

Name	Description	Web Site	Avg. $
BreatheRight	Variety of nasal strips	breatheright.com	$12 for 30
ClearPassage	Variety of nasal strips	asocorp.com/asowww/en/products/clearpassage.html	$7 for 36
Generic	Variety of nasal strips	Online and traditional drugstores have their own brands of nasal strips	$4 for 12

Nose Dilators and Clips

Name	Description	Web Site	Avg. $
Breathe EZ	Washable clip stimulates septum	breatheez.biz	$17
Breathe with EEZ	Wire band expands nostrils from inside	breathewitheez.com	$30
Nose Brace	Insert opens nostrils	nosebrace.com	$189
Nose-Caps	Nose plugs with filters	ldtgroup.com/index2.htm	$15
NoseWorks	Clip on the outside of the nose	noseworks.com/view.asp	$25
Nozovent	Clip on the outside of the nose	nosnorezone.com/accessories.html	$8
Snore Free	Clip dilates nose while magnets stimulate septum	worldofmagnets.co.uk	$15
Snore Relief ZD-100	Clip dilates nose while magnets stimulate septum	snoreremedy.us	$20

ANTI-MOUTH-BREATHING DEVICES

Name	Description	Web Site	Avg. $
Chin-Up Strips	Adhesive strips for chin to close mouth	chinupstrip.com	$13 for 30
Nose Breathe Mouthpiece for Heavy Snorer	Plastic mouthpiece promotes nose breathing, seals lips at night	nosebreathe.com	$200
Snore Guard	Plastic mouthpiece fits over lips to promote nose breathing	somni.com	$30
Snore Stopper Chin Pillow	Pillow fits around neck to keep chin up	snoringpillow.com/int	$40
Snorgon	Soft collar fits on neck to keep chin up	snorgon.com	$30
Snoring Stopper	Elastic bands fit over the head to keep mouth shut	snoringstopper.com sleepwizard.com antisnoringdevice.com	$60

ORAL APPLIANCES

Name	Description	Web Site	Avg. $
American Dental Union	Custom-fit nonprescription snoring appliance that sticks jaw out	americandentalunion.com	$200
Noiselezz Mouthpiece	Boil-and-bite clear plastic	snoring-snoring.com/view.htm	$65
PM Positioner	Positions jaw properly, through dentists	dentalservices.net	Set by DDS
The Silencer	Positions jaw properly, through dentists	the-silencer.com	Set by DDS
Sleep Pro	Two models. One is a boil-and-bite, the other a molded custom-fit device. Both stick the jaw out to open the air passageways. NOTE: Does not sell to USA yet.	sleeppro.com	$30 to $150
TheraSnore	Positions jaw properly, through dentists	distar.com/TSAppl.html	Set by DDS

CPAP Machines

Name	Description	Web Site	Avg. $
California Sleep Solutions	Online store sells CPAPs, masks, humidifiers	csscpap.com	Up to $2,000
CPAP.com	Online store sells nothing but CPAPs	cpap.com	Up to $2,000
CPAP World	Online store sells CPAPs, masks, humidifiers	cpap.net	Up to $2,000
Puritan Bennett	Manufacturer of CPAP pumps and masks	puritanbennett.com	Up to $2,000

Nasal Irrigation Systems

Name	Description	Web Site	Avg. $
NeilMed Sinus Rinse	Rinse kit (bottle and packets of salt and sodium bicarbonate) irrigates sinuses	neilmed.com	$12
SinuCleanse	Kit (bottle and salt solution packets) for gentle nasal rinse	sinucleanse.com	$15

THROAT SPRAYS AND HOMEOPATHIC CURES

Name	Description	Web Site	Avg. $
Ayr Snore Relieving Throat Spray	Natural oils lubricate throat	bfascher.com	$11
BreatheRight Snore Relief Throat Spray	Natural oils lubricate throat	breatheright.com	$12
Dr. Harris' Original Snore Formula	Natural enzymes in pill format promote better breathing	nutritionworld.com/snore	$14
Goodnight Stop Snore	Swiss mouthwash of essential oils	academyhealth.com/ goodstopsnor	$17
Helps Stop Snoring	British throat spray or gargle of eleven oils	stopsnoring.co.uk	$10 to $15
Sinus Buster	Natural pepper extract clears sinuses	sinusbuster.com	$10
SnorAway	Spray of five oils	bargainboyz.ca/snoraway	$20
SnorEase	Natural pills made of bitter orange act as decongestant	4naturalhealthherbs.com	$15

continued

THROAT SPRAYS AND HOMEOPATHIC CURES (*Continued*)

Name	Description	Web Site	Avg. $
Snoreeze	Europe's number one spray made of natural oils and vitamins	snoreeze.com	$17
SnorEnz	Fast-acting all-natural spray for instant relief, made with vitamins B_6 and E, plus peppermint	snorenz.com	$9
SnoreStop	Homeopathic chewable antisnoring tablets	snorestop.com	$7
SnoreStop Extinguisher	Homeopathic throat spray for emergency antisnoring relief	snorestop.com	$17
YSnore Spray	Homeopathic throat spray	ysnore.com	$8
YSnore Nasal Drops	Homeopathic nose drops	ysnore.com	$6

SAMPLE PRODUCTS

NEW SURGICAL PROCEDURES

Name	Description	Web Site	Avg. $
ArthroCare Corp.	Inventor and licensor of coblation, a radio frequency procedure to reduce tissues	arthrocare.com	Cost of procedure determined by doctor
Restore Medical, Inc.	Developer of Pillar System, which uses palatial inserts to stiffen upper palate	restoremedical.com	Cost of procedure determined by doctor
Somnus Medical Technologies (Gyrus Group)	Inventor and licensor of somnoplasty, using radio frequency to reduce soft palate tissues	somnoplasty.com	Cost of procedure determined by doctor

SNORE NO MORE!

ALTERNATIVE CURES

Name	Description	Web Site	Avg. $
Antisnor Therapeutic Ring	Silver ring applies acupressure to little finger of left hand	nosnor.com	$75
Breathe Easy	Herbal tea with ephedra and peppermint acts as a natural decongestant	wellfx.com	$4
I Just Want to Sleep	Exercise program to strengthen your tongue so it rests better at night	ijustwanttosleep.com	$50
MuscleToner	Straps that help you exercise and strengthen your throat muscles	snorecure.net	$80
Singing for Snorers	Three CDs and booklet teach you how to tone throat muscles by singing	singingforsnorers.com	$70

SAMPLE PRODUCTS

Name	Description	Web Site	Avg. $
Snore Stopper	Wrist bracelet shocks you into sleeping on your side when you snore	hivox-biotek.com	$100
Stop Snoring	Two CD set for self-hypnosis	wendi.com	$50
Stop Snoring Exercise Program	Exercises to improve yoursleep patterns	thestopsnoringexerciseprogram.com	$50

SNORE NO MORE!

FOR SNOREES ONLY!

Name	Description	Web Site	Avg. $
Marsona White Noise Machines	Variety of machines topump pure white noise into bedroom	earplugstore.com	$40 to $100
SilentEar Earplugs (NRR-33)	Highest-rated earplugs (NRR-33) from Israel	earplugstore.com	$10
Sleep-Eze	A plug similar to a hearing aid that masks snoring with adjustable white noise	earplugstore.com	$187
SnorePlug	Next-generation earplug—doesn't have NRR rating yet, but may be higher than NRR-33—from Taiwan	snoringshop.com	$10
Snoring Relief Kit (Earplugs)	Variety pack of eight different kinds of plugs	earplugstore.com	$18
Sound Machine Sound Soother	Twenty different white noise environments	sharperimage.com	$100

SAMPLE PRODUCTS

Name	Description	Web Site	Avg. $
White Noise CDs	One hour of soothing sounds	earplugstore.com	$9 to $25
World's Finest Ear Plugs	Moldable beeswax, cotton, and lanolin claims NRR-34	earplugsonline.com	$10 for two pair

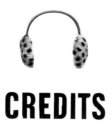

CREDITS

All original illustrations by John Rassman.

Author's photo by Larry Laszlo.

All patent illustrations courtesy of United States Patent Office.

Other photos by the author.

The illustrations and photos below are used with the permission of the following:

Page 7, "Snoring" in Semaphore,
Webster's Online Dictionary, the Rosetta Edition
(www.websters-online-dictionary.org)

Page 93, Chin Strips,
the Chin-Up Company
(www.chinupstrip.com)

Page 98, Neck Collar,
Snorgon Products,
Levin, New Zealand
(www.snorgon.com)

Pages 105, CPAP Pump and Masks,
Nellcor Puritan Bennett, Inc.
Pleasanton, California
(www.puritanbennett.com)

Page 106, Water Mask, Filipe Frade

Page 106, Native Mask, Kym Parry

Page 106, Clown, Antonio Macias

Page 123, Pillar System,
Restore Medical
(www.restoremedical.com)

Page 127, Using a Nasal Irrigation System,
NeilMed Pharmaceuticals, Inc.
(www.neilmed.com)